GW00494525

Praise for *Just Getting Started*:

'Full of advice to help us see the brighter side of this physical and mental shift.'   *Woman & Home*

'Bravo, Lisa, for lifting the veil and shifting the perspective on this season in women's lives. It's not the end but a beginning.'   JENNIFER ANISTON

'… a candid confessional'   *Psychologies*

'Your joy for life is honest and infectious, and your advice about perimenopause was a true game changer for me.'
                                                     LISA FAULKNER

'Make this your new bedside bible … Full of lived experience backed up by impeccable research, this book helped me enormously. She's my menopause Obi-Wan Kenobi and I'm so pleased she's found the time to pour everything onto the page.'   KATE THORNTON

'Lisa is a friend and mentor so when she asked me to read her book I jumped at the chance. What I wasn't prepared for was how much heart, love and light she brings to the conversation on menopause.'   MEG MATTHEWS

'Lisa and I met way back and crossing paths with her at this stage of our lives has been a blessing, as is this book. Go grab it and share it with your friends. It's an insightful look at life, menopause and beyond.' PENNY LANCASTER

'I have had the pleasure of working with Lisa and feel so privileged to call her a dear friend. She is one of the most passionate, altruistic, menopause ambassadors ... I am so proud of her and this superb book. This is another one of her achievements, helping women navigate this potentially tricky time.' DR NAOMI POTTER

'Menopause can be the scariest time of your life. This book will be your best friend and make you feel like it's the beginning, not the end.' ZOE HARDMAN

'The main lesson I've learned from Lisa is that this chapter in one's life is an opportunity for a new beginning. Change can be daunting but she teaches you how to embrace this transition with grace and curiosity.' LAUREN SANCHEZ

'Lisa's book is a reminder that while we may feel alone during menopause ... our stories are all so similar.' NAOMI WATTS

Lessons
in Life,
Love and
Menopause

Just Getting Started

Lisa Snowdon

HarperCollins*Publishers*

HarperCollins*Publishers*
1 London Bridge Street
London SE1 9GF

www.harpercollins.co.uk

HarperCollins*Publishers*
Macken House, 39/40 Mayor Street Upper
Dublin 1, D01 C9W8, Ireland

First published by HarperCollins*Publishers* 2023
This paperback edition published 2024

1 3 5 7 9 10 8 6 4 2

A catalogue record of this book is
available from the British Library

ISBN 978-0-00-860551-3

Printed and bound in the UK using 100%
renewable electricity at CPI Group (UK) Ltd

This book contains advice and information relating to healthcare. It should be
used to supplement rather than replace the advice of your doctor or another
trained health professional. If you know or suspect you have a health problem,
it is recommended that you seek your doctor's advice before embarking on any
medical programme or treatment. All efforts have been made to assure the
accuracy of the information contained in this book as of the date of publication.
This publisher and the author disclaim liability for any medical outcomes that
may occur as a result of applying the methods suggested in this book.

MIX
Paper | Supporting
responsible forestry
FSC™ C007454

This book contains FSC™ certified paper and other controlled
sources to ensure responsible forest management.

For more information visit: www.harpercollins.co.uk/green

This is to all the women in the world, the women in my life and the women who have come before me. I love you, I respect you, I see you.

I would also like to dedicate this book to my hormones, because I realise now that they have been causing chaos and disruption pretty much my whole life. (I now grant you permission to back the f*** off!)

Disclaimer

We will discuss a whole range of topics in this book. It's important for you to understand that I'm not a trained professional, and any advice that I give is just my opinion – as someone who's fascinated by, but not trained in the areas under discussion. If you want to engage with any of the therapies and services that are discussed here, make sure you always talk to a trained and accredited professional, so they can tailor their service to you. For all your health and medical needs, it's always best to speak to your GP first.

Contents

Introduction

Hi, welcome to my first ever book! It's been a long time in the making – or at least a long time in my mind – and now it's here and in your hands. So, I would like to start by giving you a big hug and thanking you from the bottom of my heart for choosing to read it.

My name is Lisa Snowdon and for the last five years I have been campaigning for better access to healthcare for women going through menopause, as well as better treatment. My own journey, which I will share with you in this book, started earlier than 'normal' and certainly earlier than I would have liked or expected, but, well, that's life – and if I have learned anything in my years in the public eye, it's that the show must go on.

I wrote this book because when I got my menopause diagnosis, I remember wishing that someone had told me what was about to happen to me. I felt lost, alone and very confused. I knew something had changed – I didn't feel like myself any more and, worse still, it was as if I was losing a big part of my identity. But for me, in that moment, there was no one to turn to. Women didn't talk freely about this period of their lives. I'm not sure why; maybe because it was too hard, or maybe because society wasn't interested or, worse, that getting old is a curse and never a blessing.

It took years before I realised that this might, among many other things, be part of our culture. And it was only after I read about Chinese medicine that I found comfort in what was happening to me. In Chinese medicine they believe that during menopause, the energy needed for our uterus, for growing a baby, becomes free to travel to the heart, generating a renewal, a rebirth, a deeper wisdom, a time for a spiritual reconnection with oneself. In other words, the menopause is time for *you*.

This is a beautiful way to express this new phase of a woman's life, and one I immediately fell in love with and that resonated with me massively. In Eastern cultures, this second spring is seen as a time to be celebrated, to be respected; it is a time of reflection – on where we have got to in our lives, where we have been, who we are, what we have achieved and where we want our life to go now. It is wonderful that wisdom and age in Asia are revered and respected. Sadly, this is so different to how ageing is viewed in Western culture.

Now I always say, 'This is the start', because that is what I believe. Menopause is not the end – far from it; it is the beginning of something truly wonderful. So, I'd like to start off by making some promises.

INTRODUCTION

In this book, I promise to be the most honest and transparent I have ever been. I will share some secrets that I have never discussed with anyone. This is my personal relationship with my hormones, with life, with getting older; from periods to pregnancy to perimenopause and now the menopause.

I promise you that whatever is around the corner, and whatever stage of the process you are at, I will show you the way. I have been through it all and I know how scary, unfamiliar and shocking this phase of your life may seem right now.

I promise that it will be OK. I was OK. You will be OK. It's going to require a lot of faith, a bit of work and a whole lot of love to get there but I, you, we *will* be OK.

My story has never been told to anyone – no magazine or journalist has ever got close to finding out what is truly inside my heart, to seeing who I really am and what my life has been. Up until this moment, I have felt that some parts of my life are private and painful – certainly too painful to share. But with you, I feel like we are friends, and I want to be raw and open, throwing caution to the wind and telling the truth, warts and all, regardless of judgement, for the first time. Of course, I would not be able to do this without the support of my wonderful partner, George (who will also feature in this book), who has helped me through some of my darkest times and been by my side at the best of times, too.

This is my story – including my mistakes, my journey and the rollercoaster that the last few years have delivered.

So, take my hand and let's walk forwards on this new, unexplored road of self-discovery and wisdom. I promise that you will feel safe, loved and supported the whole way through.

Love, Lisa x

A Personal Manual

There will be a reason why you bought this book. Perhaps it was curiosity about what the future looks like; or maybe you no longer recognise yourself and want some answers to help you deal with what is happening to you right NOW. Perhaps you have lost that precious connection with someone you love dearly who may be experiencing some of these things and you want to learn a little more about how to reconnect with them. This can only be done with understanding, empathy and support. Three simple words that could truly change your life.

In the last few years, I have seen a real shift in attitude towards women going through the menopause, and while we still have a long way to go, I am grateful to my peers – people like Mariella Frostrup, Meg Mathews, Davina McCall, Dr Naomi Potter, Kate Codrington, Carolyn Harris MP, all the women involved in the Menopause Mandate and Naomi Watts to name a few – for shining a bright light on this subject. I do urge you to read as much as you can to get the best possible overview; I will add a list of some of my favourite books at the end, but if this is the first book you're reading on the subject, it's a good start. Or maybe you've read them all and are looking for more information or another point of view.

As I have gone into the menopause, I have come to realise that there just isn't enough support for all women in this situation. I don't think this is right, which is why I have been campaigning alongside some friends and many passionate women for better healthcare and access to life-changing treatments during this key time in our lives. Along the way I have met and learned from many experts in their respective fields, and I have asked them to contribute their thoughts to this book, so within these pages you'll find their advice, which I hope you'll find useful and informative.

Whatever your reason for picking up this book, welcome! I hope the following chapters will provide some comfort, direction and answers for you. I hope it will help lift your spirits, calm your mind and make you smile from time to time. I hope it will be your road map as you navigate this new path.

As with any road less travelled, the first step is always the hardest, so, for ease, I have set this book up in several parts:

PART ONE: WE'RE GOING THROUGH CHANGES

I will start with a detailed account of what was happening to me when I first noticed major changes. I didn't really know what was happening, so things like mood swings, feeling low, sudden outbursts, skin changes and weight gain were very confusing. Like so many women, I was misdiagnosed and left to try to find my way through all on my own.

This all started in my early forties, and it took a good eight years to finally pinpoint that it was perimenopause. As I write this in my kitchen, as a 51-year-old woman, I can confirm to you that I am now definitely post-menopausal, meaning that I dealt with my perimenopausal years without the correct advice, help and support that every woman deserves. So, I want to look back and revisit my younger years to examine my relationship with my hormones going from puberty to adult life. I feel it's important to address this now to form a full picture of what we go through as women in our lifetimes.

Perimenopause is a key element of our journey as women and plays a huge part for most of us, so I will talk about all the symptoms – the more common ones and the sneaky little less common ones – to give you an idea of what might be to come for you. One of the hardest facts I had to face up to was the possibility of never having children. This, in particular, was difficult to write, as there are still moments where it can throw me off – especially when I am asked live on TV or in interviews: 'Have you come to terms with not having children?' In that moment it feels as though the air has been sucked out of the room, or a scab has been ripped off, because it's never as simple as people think. It's extremely personal and I will, for the first time, explain why and how I managed to overcome this.

PART TWO: EYE OF THE STORM

One of the biggest lessons I have learned in life is that it's not the destination but how you get there. In order to get to the highs, we have to go through the lows, and my goodness did the lows come thick and fast! As I started to feel the effects of perimenopause, and in particular the changes in mood, I realised I was experiencing a lot of unresolved negativity, suppressed emotions and unprocessed trauma (particularly surrounding my relationships with men). It was important that I addressed all this in order to protect my self-esteem and self-confidence, enabling me to move into a place of acceptance of getting older without being afraid of the future and googling how to bedazzle your Zimmer frame.

It was obvious that my metabolism was slowing down, my hormone levels were fluctuating and the weight just started piling on. The good news here is that there is help, and the simplest solution is that we need to move more, so I will go through the activities that helped me most – and I promise it will be more fun than an SAS training boot camp, which, to be fair, might not be saying much.

Regardless, the reason I am keen to get you moving is because in doing so you'll feel more positive, and you will hopefully see impacts in every area of your life. What it did for me was to give me a renewed sense of self-worth and confidence, both of which were vital in helping me to realise that the best friend I ever needed was me. Friendships are important, there's no denying it, but during my perimenopause years I had to re-evaluate some of my connections. In particular, I had to learn to listen to my intuition with regards to how some people made me feel; and to honour and protect myself I had to make do without certain people in my life.

Working on ourselves is the biggest project we'll ever be a part of, and it's in this time that we have to start putting ourselves at the top of the priority list. That's not to say it's easy work, and it can sometimes be very tiring. We need to simplify our lives and try to eliminate some of the unnecessary stress – whether in the form of people, work, your love life, etc. – because perimenopause and menopause bring sleepless nights. You can find yourself waking up sometimes three times a night, and with each new day just putting one foot in front of the other can be a challenge. We have to conserve our energy and truly look after ourselves in order to get to the light. And speaking of light, there was one at the end of the tunnel for me, which came in the form of life-changing, beloved HRT – hormone replacement therapy – or, HR sweet T, to you and me.

PART THREE: WE'RE JUST GETTING STARTED

And that, ladies, leads me to Part Three – my favourite part – which refers to you and me, and the fact that, well, we're just getting started. I can honestly say that by living my life in a mindful way and by being present and practising gratitude, I am pretty fucking happy with what I have got. I am definitely a glass is half full kind of girl, and I really recommend that you start to use this mantra, too; because life is short, and as long as you have your health and love around you – in any form you find it – it will all be OK.

Speaking of love, after searching high and low for my missing libido, I can report that I found it. It's a little less sparky than it used to be (I am not going to lie), but I have included a whole section of tips, tricks and advice on getting your jiggy back. Another thing that will help you with your confidence is noticing the changes in your skin when you take better, more focused care of your nutrition

– because what you put inside you can help you glow outwardly, so I will share a few of my secret recipes for doing just that.

This is your time to shine and do all the things you have ever wanted to do – take that trip of a lifetime, book that spa retreat, go backpacking around Asia, enjoy guilt-free you time. You deserve it, you've earned it. For me, it was travel, but for you it can be whatever you've put away to the back of your mind.

Here we go, hold on tight.

Part One

We're Going Through Changes

HORMONES

So, hormones. I mean, like, wtf? They have been the bane of my existence my whole life, kicking around in the background and sometimes goddamn taking over and causing chaos for what seems to me like for ever.

I was quite a late developer; well, that's what my mum always said. I was painfully thin and bullied for it for most of my days in high school. It seemed to me that puberty had passed me by, and when all the other girls' bodies were changing, mine stayed the same, frozen in time. I used to lie in the bath at night, looking down at my childlike body, with its little gnat-bite nipples, and pray for my boobs to grow and my body to develop. It felt as if every girl in my class had started their period years before me and I was so self-conscious; I desperately wanted mine to start, too. It consumed me so much, making me very unhappy; I put a silly, unhealthy amount of pressure on myself for such a young person – and so unnecessarily – but I really did feel like there was something wrong with me.

My mum had taught me about the birds and bees at a young age, around seven or eight. I remember it like it was yesterday. She was in the bath, me sitting next to her and listening to her explain how babies were made, and telling me that I would, at some point, start my periods. I felt incredibly grown up to have been privy to this extremely adult conversation and thought it must mean that I would soon encounter all that she was telling me.

Perhaps that's why I put pressure on myself for it all to happen as quickly as possible. However, it took almost another seven or eight years before I did get my first period. Yes, you've done the maths ... I was sixteen. Looking back now, I know I was actually very fortunate, as some of the girls in my class started theirs when they were as young as ten or eleven, but at the time I was so envious of them – surely they were women now? I now think that is too young an age to have to grow up, to deal with that level of respon- sibility, pain and discomfort, not to mention embarrassment at gym time or swimming classes. It's so unfair – you are still just a kid. Back then, though, because I did not feel part of this 'grown-up club', I was so self-conscious. In every human biology class, I was convinced that the very hand- some Mr Wright (who I think we all had a huge crush on) would ask us to raise our hands and say who had started their periods and I would have to lie, but then I wouldn't have any information about how it felt because it wasn't true. I mean, like that was ever going to happen! But the bottom line is that when I eventually started, I felt my life had really begun and I was now going to be accepted into every friendship group – including the mean kids' group.

Reflecting on my life, I realise that my hormones have ruled and controlled me, as dramatic as that sounds, running a rollercoaster of emotions and feelings that weren't my own – like an alien invasion of my body. They seriously have a lot to answer for, and I am sure you will be able to relate, whatever your age. I felt the turbulence they caused each month in varying degrees – manifesting in sadness, irritability, anger, emotional outbursts, crippling anxiety – and some days I really did not like who I was or recognise myself at all. And this went on for years, way beyond my adolescence.

The irony is not lost on me that I ended up working as a model in my first job, when clearly, I already had issues with my body image. I would look in the mirror and the body dysmorphia would be so real and so illogically terrifying that I didn't want to leave the house, let alone turn up to work on a photoshoot where I would be working with strangers, wearing clothes that weren't mine and which quite possibly wouldn't fit me, due to my swollen and water-retentive body. I knew I would be scrutinised on set, having been primped and preened and squeezed into the tiny sample sizes swinging from the stylists' rail, experiencing feelings of horror and dread in the knowledge that I would have to dig deep and deliver somehow.

I realise now, I can recognise that is perhaps where my deep-rooted issues of imposter syndrome stemmed from – the worry of never being enough and of being turned away from shoots as I didn't look like my model card or ad in person; that I wasn't good enough, pretty enough, slim enough. Now this wasn't every day, of course, and I did have some incredible clients who I worked with repeatedly. We travelled all over the world together and had the best time, and I look back on these moments fondly, as they were some of my favourites over my modelling career. The scary, intimidating times came in Paris and Milan, where work was very serious, and the agents and the clients could be very mean. On occasion, I would be told to go home from shoots because clothes didn't fit me, often because my breasts were too big for the tiny size-zero clothes. I was told to lose weight multiple times, which I wasn't happy about. Having been such a skinny kid and bullied for that, it just didn't sit well with me that now that I had developed into the woman I had longed to be, and finally, my little gnat bites had grown (be careful what you wish for, kids), I was being told I didn't fit in there either. That sense of not being welcome or good enough continued into my twenties. And when you are told something enough times, you do start to believe it.

I don't blame the industry exactly; it's just how fashion works – seasons change, different body shapes are in or out. Obviously, these days designers are so much more aware and conscious of inclusivity, but back then, most seasons it was about models having superhuman body shapes and being long and lean clothes horses for designers to hang their creations on.

Nothing looked good on me at this time of the month, and I would literally go through every item in my wardrobe in despair, as ridiculous as that sounds, the anxiety and dislike for myself being so real. If I am honest, I only truly felt like myself for about five days each month, usually when I started to bleed – then I would feel relief washing over me that a) I wasn't pregnant, and b) that I would not be a slave to my hormones for just a few days. I was lucky, as I didn't struggle with too much pain or cramps – at least, nothing that a few painkillers couldn't handle – instead experiencing some bloating, breast tenderness and pimples, not only around my chin but also on my butt. (Does anyone else suffer with those? Very embarrassing, and quite frankly, painful. And when picked they scar … be warned.)

The rise and fall of my hormone levels throughout those twenty-eight-day cycles – in particular progesterone, a hormone I now know that I, like many women, am extremely sensitive to – called the shots and dictated my moods for thirty years, making me moody, grumpy, angry, agitated and hungry, always craving chocolate and sweet treats. It was a real yo-yo of emotions.

Testosterone was also a key factor, and now it has upped and left my body, leaving my libido pretty much on the floor. This is the complete opposite to who I was as a young woman, when my sex drive went through the roof from month to month, as the rise of this hormone caused a surge of yearning, sometimes taking me over, causing me to make silly mistakes with men. When I look back, I definitely blame the surges and changes happening in my body.

I speak with lots of younger women who struggle with anxiety and sadness throughout the month, just as I did. We were never taught at school about the potential impact of our cycles on our mental health; there was no focus on the problems we might encounter – we were just left to work it all out on our own.

Hormones, weirdly, are never considered by anyone – even professionals – to be the issue when we are struggling; they are not ever at the top of the list of potential contributing factors to our state of mind or body issues. Our hormones are clever and like to trick us with their lack of consistency and their rebellious attitude. They have the power to create a storm within, and it's all beyond our control.

I know now only too well the anguish caused by the fluctuation of the levels in my body, affecting so many areas of my health, and this is something that I think we should all be talking more about, and from an earlier age.

But I also think we should be starting the conversation much sooner about what happens *after* our fertile years.

The menopause can – and will – affect everyone in diverse ways; Dr Nighat Arif, a very well-known and respected NHS doctor, told me that some women of colour don't think it can happen to them, and that it's just for white people. That is a measure of how undereducated we have all been when it comes to this. But menopause is not just a white middle-class person's problem – it affects all women of all races and cultures.

Thankfully, the word perimenopause is on the radar now, but when I was going through it that word was rarely used. The menopausal woman also looked quite different to me; she was much older, she was frail, she was using a walking stick or walker, she had a head full of grey hair. It all seemed so far off into the future that I couldn't possibly contemplate that it was happening to me.

We are, unfortunately, still a way off getting the help we need, as many doctors still don't understand perimeno-pause symptoms. If a woman in her early to mid-forties goes to her doctor complaining of low mood, low libido and stiff, aching joints, it's not often picked up as a hormone issue or possibly early perimenopause symp-toms.

Our hormones are so up and down through the month, and indeed through our lives, the only constant being the confusion they leave us in. It is extremely distressing, and as you enter adulthood and think you finally have a handle on it, you get whooped around the head with more change. Let me warn you: this rollercoaster continues into menopause. The little hormone disruptors fuck shit up.

SIGNS AND SYMPTOMS OF THE PERIMENOPAUSE AND MENOPAUSE

I have been very open publicly about my journey these last few years, and in particular what I have been through. The reason is because, put simply, I wanted to start the conversation about the changes I was experiencing, as there just wasn't enough information out there to help *me*. So, before we go any further, let's discuss key signs you should be looking out for that will indicate that you might be in perimenopause or menopause.

Currently there are around sixty verified signs and symptoms associated with the perimenopause and the menopause, and doctors are still counting more every day – by the time this goes to print, who knows, that number may be closer to a hundred!

Every day, a new symptom or side effect is linked to this time in our life, not just the more well-known ones like hot flushes and periods stopping. In fact, referring to periods stopping is a bit misleading, as you can still be having regular bleeds each month but be very much perimenopausal, experiencing other effects, which is why it is so important to highlight all the changes, so we can be on top of our health.

The good news is that we are unlikely to suffer with all these symptoms – otherwise life would be hell on earth! Although, speaking from experience, even a few can wreak absolute havoc, leaving you fraught with anxiety. The sleep deprivation, too, is unbearable and makes many women feel that life is not worth living. The menopause can also cause relationships to break down and some women leave their jobs, due to sudden panic attacks, anxiety, lack of confidence and feelings of being judged and/or being invisible, feeling they are no longer competent to carry on.

I have felt like this some days, and it is the loneliest place to be – not recognising who you are, not understanding the changes. You feel like you are losing your mind. I've had days when I didn't sleep and had to be at work, and I honestly felt so out of sorts – almost like I was having an out-of-body experience, not even knowing my own name. Feeling that way, working in mostly live TV, meant that my job was a huge struggle. There have been days when I didn't want to get out of bed. I wanted the duvet to swallow me up and the world around me to disappear. I hated who I was and how I was thinking. I hated life. I didn't trust myself not to make mistakes, and had no faith in myself. I had also put on weight, which exacerbated my confidence issues, not least because people had started to notice and were sending me mean messages and comments on my social media.

I had just got back together with George, after a fifteen-year break, and was the happiest in that relationship that I had ever been. There were weeks of blissful happiness, and we certainly loved spending all our time together (we moved in together immediately), and in my heart I knew, after all these years, that he was the one. He was kind, loving and fun to be around, but still I felt myself trying to push him away. I was vile towards him and used him as an emotional punchbag, unsure of who I was or what I was turning into. I have since come to understand that the trauma from past relationships had left me suspicious, hurt and vulnerable. I was scared – actually, terrified – of letting someone in, someone who I knew in my heart wanted to love me for me and who only had pure intentions (a rarity in my career world), but the timing was terrible, with hormones raging, as well as my moods.

I don't know if I could have been as honest as I am about my journey through perimenopause and menopause if I hadn't been with George. Who knows? I've always been a girl's girl and I'm always candid about what I'm feeling and what I'm going through. In my head, I was stuck in the old way of thinking that the menopause signified old age, of not being attractive to the opposite sex, and not feeling wanted or valid. I was so lucky and had support from a fantastic man who has been championing me for ever. I feel so fortunate that he came back into my life at this time; thankfully, this man won't be pushed away, no matter what.

I do understand that's not the case for everyone, though, which is why I also believe there should be support groups for men dealing with their partners at this time. Husbands, uncles, brothers, sons – the entire male population – are lost at this tricky time and don't know how to communicate with the women in their lives. The taboo surrounding this topic is thankfully starting to disappear, so the conversation can now be opened across all genders. And it's about bloody time, as it's taken years and years and years of women suffering in silence, feeling embarrassed, ashamed and confused about what is happening to them, to get to this point.

Now I must caveat all this by saying that not every woman experiences unpleasant symptoms; some people sail through this. It's just that, for me, it wasn't like that. I didn't know what was happening to me and thought there was something seriously wrong. I can see that at the start of my forties was when things started to get bad. But because I was only around forty-two years old, doctors didn't put two and two together and work out that there could be a slight hormone imbalance, and that it could be down to the perimenopause. I am just as guilty here, as I didn't know either. However, it all makes sense to me after the research I have done over the last five years, knowing that our fertility starts to be challenged in our late thirties and early forties.

PERIMENOPAUSE

If you aren't quite there yet, or you think you might be heading that way soon, the first thing I'd like to say about perimenopause is that it isn't something to be fearful of. So please, don't be scared to investigate it; when it does hit you, you'll be so glad you read up about it, as being aware of how things might change for you is really the best preparation there is.

We have oestrogen receptors all over our bodies, from the roots of our hair down to the tips of our toes, which means that symptoms can vary hugely from person to person, affecting any area of the body, too.

So, as I said, there are roughly sixty symptoms that we know about at the moment. You might be familiar with the more typical ones, such as hot flushes/flashes and night sweats, as well as erratic cycles or no periods at all, but there are also many lesser-known symptoms, meaning that women are suffering and struggling for longer than they need to because they don't recognise or register that how they are feeling is hormone-related.

For me, not knowing anything at all about what was heading my way was the worst. There were moments when I thought I was losing my mind, and that was scary.

When you know what is going on, it's much easier to make changes and understand what you need to do to make life easier.

My perimenopause crept up on me out of nowhere, and as I've just said, the scariest part was not being able to identify the changes and what was causing them. I could put so many of the symptoms down to something else, but once I began to understand that this was not just a one- or two-day phase, it dawned on me that something was happening that wasn't linked to just a bad night's sleep, a hangover or a dodgy meal.

Having to go through perimenopause in silence, so to speak, has made me passionate about raising awareness and being open with what's happening to us. Half the battle with perimenopause is not recognising yourself and not understanding what's happening. For so many years, women have had to suffer in silence, ashamed of this change in their bodies, their hormones and their mental state. For me, that's not acceptable, and I now feel so positive about the changes I've gone through that I am determined to spread the word; we must talk about this on a daily basis and shout it from the rooftops, until everybody gets it, until there are menopause policies in place in every workplace and menopause specialists in every GP surgery, and until children understand what's happening to their teachers, their grandmas or even their mums. That's when I'll feel that it is no longer a taboo subject.

MY PERIMENOPAUSE DIAGNOSIS

Women can go for years being misdiagnosed or wrongly prescribed medication when it's quite clear that what they are going through is the start of perimenopause. So many women I have spoken to have been fobbed off with random medication and not appropriately looked after for as long as ten years, effectively losing those vital years as their health deteriorates.

At my first doctor's appointment I was prescribed anti-depressants as a first line of attack. It didn't sit well with me, and I remember being incredibly angry when the doctor suggested them as I just knew that something else was going on – that something had fundamentally changed in me. The waves of sadness that enveloped me from time to time did not feel like me. And I was right. It was something else – it was the perimenopause starting to kick in. Yes, I was at my wits' end; yes, I broke down at the doctor's appointment; yes, I guess it may have seemed like I was having an emotional breakdown and antidepressants were what sprang to mind for my doctor. But the bottom line is, this happens to so many of us – we don't know what is happening and nor do the doctors (correction, not all doctors), so it's down to us to research more about our hormones and other options of what could be happening to us to ensure that we are able to navigate our appointments more easily. Armed with this information, we can make suggestions and take along our checklist of signs and symptoms, so that we stand a chance of getting a correct diagnosis.

Not knowing any better at the time, however, I took the antidepressants. They were selective serotonin reuptake inhibitors (SSRIs) and I went on taking them for roughly six months. I continued to struggle most days, being a total bitch to George for no reason at all, my symptoms changing somewhat along the way – because that is the other thing with perimenopause: from month to month new symptoms crop up just to confuse us and our loved ones even more. It wasn't until around two years later that a friend, the incredible Sarah Bradden, gave me an answer for what was going on. Sarah is the most wonderful healer, working in Chinese medicine, acupuncture, reiki and reflexology. She was the first person to identify that my hormones were out of sync. Every time I used to see her for an appointment I was on my knees – overly emotional, wrought with exhaustion, puffy and swollen – and each time, she would look at my tongue (this is how Chinese medicine determines the overall health of a person) and declare 'you are getting your period'. Well, she was right, and I would literally start bleeding the next day. With each one of her needles going in, I felt a sense of relief, almost like the air being released from a balloon. Tears would stream down my cheeks, and I'd feel a wonderful sense of peace and calm. My swollen and unhappy body soothed, I would leave there floating, determined to hang on to that sensation of zen.

Sarah was convinced I was perimenopausal and recommended I see a private hormone doctor on Harley Street. I was beyond happy to finally be able to almost identify what was wrong with me, and thrilled at a solid recommendation, so I booked the appointment and off I went. After blood tests and ultrasounds of my ovaries, I was packed off and told to come back for the results. Already, it had cost me around £1,000 and I knew coming back for my results would require booking and paying for yet another appointment. The doctor was a strange little man, doddering around, mumbling to himself, but I had been told he was good, so I persevered. I went back to get my results thinking that there was no way I was in the perimenopause, but as I sat there opposite him, he delivered the news I hadn't been expecting: I was indeed perimenopausal. But rather than leave it there or offer sympathy or support, he said, so this means you're getting old, there is no denying it, and you most definitely cannot have children.

His words winded me. I remember digging my nails into my hands, squeezing so hard it felt like I had drawn blood, trying my hardest to not cry. Maybe I was being too sensitive, but the lump in my throat and the pain I was causing myself digging my dagger-sharp nails into my hands helped to stop the tears and instead I just nodded and said I understood, that's fine.

I went to another private doctor after another recommendation (I am not in any way blaming my friends, as they were really happy with these doctors), but they just didn't work for me either. I did not get them or their way of assessing feminine health at all. He suggested I book into the aesthetic facialist upstairs for some 'anti-ageing treatments and injectables'. I mean, really? Completely unethical and, quite frankly, rude. Plus, he prescribed progesterone cream exactly like the previous doctor, not oestrogen, which I now know is exactly what is needed. I have since learned that we don't absorb progesterone through the skin and that it is better taken either orally or vaginally, as I now take it, due to my progesterone sensitivity.

Anyway, I didn't last long with this doctor either, for obvious reasons, but finally, with doctor number three, I struck gold. Welcome to the party, the incredible Dr Naomi Potter! If you follow me on social media, you will know that for the last few years we have set up a weekly chat on our page, open to everyone, discussing the ins and outs of perimenopause and menopause. It is called Midweek Menopause Madness. On this, as the name suggests, we unpick the madness of this time in our lives. It has not only helped me to understand more, but I know it has helped my community, too.

Naomi has changed my life. I adore her, and I will forever be indebted to her for her help, continued guidance, knowledge and expertise, and I am thrilled to say that she has become a very close friend. Her practice and her associates at Menopause Care are fantastic. It is a private practice, but I think it is worth every penny.

WHAT TO EXPECT

The perimenopause and the menopause are just moments of transition in a woman's life. In the simplest terms, it is a time when our ovaries stop producing the levels of hormones that they did in our teenage years and up. I would compare perimenopause to your worst-ever PMT/ PMS. You feel like a ***** from hell. I know I've had moments when I felt myself go a little bit mad and had to remind myself that it's not me, it's my hormones. One thing I can confidently say is that perimenopause is a moving target; just when you think you've got it under control, something else comes into the mix and whoops your arse all over again. But the good news is that things do improve, and, in time, you will begin to feel more human again.

So, what should you expect when perimenopause strikes? This is how it was for me:

Mood

The low mood and bouts of depression that hit me as I entered perimenopause were completely out of character, and because I was younger than most people when this happened, I didn't put two and two together to work out that this could all be down to a hormone imbalance.

Changing periods

I started to bleed often, almost haemorrhaging. Some days, I would bleed through my clothes almost immediately after changing my tampon. I have never seen that amount of blood and clots, and that worried me a lot. The cramps and the pain caused nausea that was sometimes so bad I thought I had food poisoning, and couldn't get out of bed.

Anger

While both George and I still did not know what was happening, we were trying to navigate around my awful temper, with all my bursts of rage directed at him. Always him. George took the brunt of my anger every time, especially when I was in a dark mood. My volatile, quite nasty outbursts would come out of the blue – totally unpredictable, for me and for him. After the event, I would feel the most awful guilt, which would stay with me for days, the aftershocks of the outbursts rocking me and my conscience. There were times when I felt it would break me.

On a related note, I also found that I couldn't drink wine, because I knew that would make me react in spiteful ways. I later found out that this was because wine was causing a histamine reaction, which results in the body not being able to process sugars which can impact our behaviour. You'll be happy to know that I can responsibly enjoy a nice glass or two these days, now that I am through the other side!

Weight gain
My weight started to creep up and up, and it kept going until I was around three stone heavier than I wanted to be.

Hot flushes
Pretty soon I started having hot flushes. Again, these would come out of nowhere and cause me embarrassment and complete panic. I literally felt like someone had set me on fire.

Brain fog
My brain started to fail me not long after I entered perimenopause. I would regularly forget names and feel somewhat foggy and confused from time to time. In addition, I would suffer from anxiety, and I still do. It would get so bad that I didn't want to leave the house, preferring to stay at home and say no to work coming in – particularly if it was something that would push me out of my comfort zone. As I mentioned before, I have always had imposter syndrome, but now it would rear its ugly head to the point where I wanted to pack work in altogether – even the day-to-day job

that I love on *This Morning* and other exciting presenting opportunities that should have been joyful. I didn't trust myself to do a good job and started to feel as if I had no idea what I was doing. I didn't trust my brain any more.

Sleep

The night-time hot flushes left me with many a sleepless night. The bed would be soaking wet – like, soaking – and to get through the night I would have to lay down lots of towels to try to absorb it, but then the chill of the cold, damp towels would keep me shivering throughout the night. It was always the same pattern: hot, cold, hot, cold. George nicknamed me the Furnace; my body temperature was out of control, and I couldn't regulate it at all.

I would be exhausted each night falling into bed, and would do all the things I knew would help me to wind down to try to get a good night's sleep: I would listen to Deepak Chopra, use my pillow sprays and take my magnesium. I would get into bed feeling like I had control of it all, then, just as I was falling asleep, the adrenaline would take over, seizing my heart in a vice-like grip, causing me to panic and feel like I was dying. Then, to make it all worse, I'd have to get up and go to pee. Every hour. How I still had any liquid left in my body to pee through the night, I still have no idea.

These nights were the worst and the longest. Every morning, I would feel like a shadow of myself, unable to function and scared to go out into the world. Just putting one foot in front of the other seemed a terrifying prospect.

These are just some of the symptoms that I experienced, but as I have said, there are so many, so let's start at the top and work down a list of the most common ones and see which you can relate to:

- Brain fog
- Anxiety
- Panic attacks
- Low mood and depression
- Mood swings
- Anger/rages
- Being over-emotional
- Inability to process stress
- Sadness
- Feeling out of control
- Headaches
- Migraines
- Memory loss
- Lack of concentration
- Lack of self-confidence
- Hair loss
- Tinnitus
- Eyesight changes
- Vertigo
- Skin changes, including dry, itchy skin

WE'RE GOING THROUGH CHANGES

- Sore gums
- Teeth moving
- Mouth ulcers
- Burning mouth
- Dry mouth
- Metallic taste in the mouth
- Stiff neck
- Frozen shoulder
- Aching joints and muscles
- Hot flushes
- Night sweats
- Heart palpitations
- No energy
- Weight gain
- Weight loss
- Difficulty sleeping
- Vaginal dryness
- Lack of libido
- Having to pee often
- Bad body odour
- PMS-like symptoms
- Breast tenderness
- Inability to regulate body temperature
- Chills
- IBS-like symptoms
- Irregular periods
- Heavy periods

I would encourage you to write down a list of the symptoms you are experiencing (or print out the above), then make an appointment with your doctor immediately, regardless of your age, to discuss how you will go forwards and start to feel like you again. Do not be afraid to discuss anything with the doctor; nothing is off limits. I promise you cannot embarrass them as there is nothing they haven't heard before. So throw it all out there, but if you find anything too awkward (perhaps vaginal dryness or irritable bowel, for example), just hand them a list of those more sensitive symptoms.

FERTILITY

When I think of menopause in the general sense, and certainly when I was younger and heard the word spoken, my mind would immediately go to a time when women can no longer have children. This was all I ever equated it with. For me, when that moment came, I knew I had to be strong. Although the majority of women have had children by the time they get to this stage, some will enter the menopause early, before they have had a chance to do so, which makes this experience very different and brings up a whole host of emotions. So, I want to take some time to explain how my situation has affected my own life and journey.

Pretty much my whole adult life I have been judged for not having a family, whether by the industry I work in, through casual comments from confused mums or by society in general. But as with everything, the biggest pressure is that which we put on ourselves, and I could always subliminally feel that biological clock ticking in the background without anyone having to tell me or ask me about children.

It can be hard for those of us who haven't become a parent, perhaps through choice or other reasons, to not feel judged or misunderstood by others, or, worse, like we have failed in life. The crazy thing is, I always dreamed of having children; I have felt maternal ever since I can remember, and thinking back to when I was a little girl, that was my main ambition in life – my only vision for my future was to be a mum of two little ones. I had this dream that I wanted my first child to be a boy, so he could be the older, protective brother for his younger sister.

I was a child of the 70s, when most women around me were housewives, so I wasn't exactly inspired to have a career. I am the eldest of three girls, with a ten-year age gap between myself and my youngest sister. When she arrived, pretty much out of the blue, it seemed to me, she was the perfect real-life doll for me to play with. I would walk her in her pushchair, dress her up and feel so proud when people would stop me to exclaim how cute she was. I was convinced they thought she was mine. I would check on her constantly while she slept, making sure she was still breathing, helping to feed and change her. To this day, we are still very close, and I adore her. In fact, I adore both of my sisters and feel extremely maternal towards them.

My mum and dad separated when I was around sixteen, which was obviously hard but also a huge wake-up call for us all. I had to be more adult at home, while also dealing with seeing our parents going through pain and heartache. For me, it also highlighted for the first time that marriage as an institution maybe wasn't all it was cracked up to be, something I now know to have had a significant impact on me, shaping my thoughts about future relationships.

It was my mum who instigated the split, and in an unconventional move she left the family home, so that we were raised by my dad. Dad thought it best for us to stay in the house we had lived in up until then and carry on going to the same school, so as not to unsettle us any more than was necessary. He was trying to make it easier for us all. He did a stellar job with me and my sisters, and I have the utmost respect for him. He continued to work long, hard hours, holding down his job in London, commuting every day, and he had to acquire cooking skills literally overnight. I guess he had to shape up – and quick. It was a tricky time for us all, but maybe more for my younger sisters, as I was almost grown up and could escape home life in the usual ways that teenagers do, by going out and getting drunk with my mates.

In the beginning, I thought the decision my mum made was extremely selfish and cold, and I blamed her – I didn't understand. Over the years, I've worked very hard on every aspect of my life, and this one is no different. I've done a lot of soul-searching and tried many different therapies, including some past-life regression and hypnotherapy, to try to let go of the blame and anger I felt at her departure.

The reason I am talking about my parents and the decisions they made is because these early experiences have had an impact on my own relationships. I don't want to be judgemental like I used to be when I was younger, trying to point the finger and blame people for the hurt and disappointment I felt. I have come to respect my mum's decision, because in the end it was harder for her to leave us than it was to stay. She had to really dig deep and completely turn her life inside out to make that decision. I now think it was an extremely brave thing to do, to change her life as dramatically as she did. It has taken many years, but if I put myself in my mum's shoes and realise the pain she went through to leave her children, I can see that as a mother, it is never an easy choice. She was so young when she had me (my parents were seventeen and eighteen); it takes a huge amount of maturity and dedication to raise a family, and it's hard when you're barely an adult yourself.

One day, Mum and I had a heart-to-heart and I found out that her childhood was a very unhappy one. It was a difficult conversation for both of us, but I strongly encourage everyone to have open and honest chats with their loved ones (if they can) to try to understand things from their point of view. It broke my heart to hear about her struggles, but it has helped me to understand why she is the way she is and why she did what she did. I have a beautiful relationship with both my mum and dad now, and I adore them more than anything in this world.

My family story is very common; relationships break down and many marriages don't work out. It's the reality of life – people change and grow apart, some people were never meant to be together in the first place, some just fall into relationships and some, however hard they try, cannot make their relationships work. We are all doing the best we possibly can with the life we have been given. We don't get a manual; we don't get any help or advice on how to be the best children, the best parents or the best partners and friends. People make mistakes – we all fuck up occasionally.

If you are reading this and it is bringing up emotions, my heart goes out to you. I truly hope that me being so open about how my personal situation changed and shaped me helps you to put some feelings to bed, figure stuff out and try some therapy to deal with your pain or any other emotions you are experiencing.

From someone who isn't a parent, I can still see how difficult it is to raise a child and how challenging and exhausting it can be. Sometimes we just need to be kinder to everybody around us, especially to our loved ones, and to manage our expectations about how we think others should be doing things. Kindness is everything; understanding is everything.

Nevertheless, it is a sad situation when your parents break up and I do think it has contributed to some of the feelings I have had of not being enough – that lack of self-worth – something I know that many children with divorced or separated parents feel. It's the constant thought that maybe I could have done something to have changed the situation, perhaps been a better daughter or a different person altogether. I also know that it significantly impacted how I felt about relationships and having children – my barriers went up and, unbeknown to me, I purposely attracted and sought out the wrong type of man. Perhaps subconsciously, I knew they couldn't hurt me because they would never be in my life long enough anyway. They weren't the marrying kind, or faithful, loving or loyal, and that suited me, because I could be in control. I thought that was what I wanted. But how wrong I was. Thinking about the relationships I had when I was much younger now and imagining myself with one of those men has made it much easier for me to process these errors of judgement (rather than beat myself up about them) as I realise it would never have worked.

So when it came to the idea of becoming a mother, the simple fact is, time just ran out. Coming from a separated family, I always knew that I wanted any union I entered into to be unbreakable, solid. That was more important to me than having a baby on my own; I preferred to wait to find my forever, not realising that would mean there would be other sacrifices. It is unbelievable to me how quickly time has passed. All the while I was trying to figure myself out, and then suddenly it was too late.

I sometimes think it's easier if we all believe in fate: what is meant to be will be; what is meant to be yours you will get, and what is not will pass you by. But it is not always so straightforward.

The truth is, I have been pregnant twice.

The first time, I knew I was pregnant straight away. I was in my late twenties, and I had just come back from a holiday with a boyfriend. I remember that I was on the contraceptive pill, but there was one night on this trip when I was sick. Now, I don't recall if I drank too much or if it was food poisoning, but I do remember as I stood at the mirror two weeks later, my breasts tender and sore, thinking that perhaps that was the night I could have conceived and I should have taken extra precautions. My body immediately felt different. I remember expressing my concern to my then boyfriend – to be honest, I am not sure he was even listening, but either way he didn't really seem very bothered. I also remember that back then you went to the doctor to find out if you were pregnant. I booked myself an appointment, expecting my boyfriend to come with me, but I ended up going alone. That was a warning sign, and it was like a kick in the guts. I think I'd already made my mind up on my way to the surgery, knowing in my heart, given that he couldn't even be bothered to come to the first doctor's appointment with me, the kind of father he would be.

Sure enough, the doctor confirmed my suspicions; I was very much pregnant. I went home feeling pretty numb and confused. I expected my boyfriend to at least be downstairs, awaiting my arrival, maybe on the edge of his seat, ready to hear the news. But he wasn't. There was no sign of life. It was eerily quiet, even though it was late, some time after lunch. I went upstairs and found this guy still passed out asleep. It truly broke my heart that he was so unconcerned about how I was, how I had got on and whether or not we were going to be having a baby together. I just couldn't believe the nerve of him, still asleep in my house without a care. I knew in that moment that I did not want to bring a child into this world and one day have to explain to them why I wasn't with their father and what kind of man he was. I felt such disappointment and betrayal; he clearly had no sense of responsibility and didn't care about me. I knew that I couldn't be connected to him for the rest of my life, and it made the decision easier for me to not only end the relationship, but also have a termination. My mum came with me to the local clinic in my area. It wasn't a nice experience, nor one I was happy about, but I did feel very strong in my resolve and knew that it was the right decision for me.

Every now and then I think about that baby, even more so now that I can't have kids and have left it too late to start a family. That little boy or little girl would be very much grown up – would they have been a dancer or a performer, a teacher, a writer or a trainspotter? These 'what-ifs' can be all-consuming, and I still experience guilt, shame and disappointment that I chose to do that. In my darkest moments, I blame myself for choosing to end a life, which leaves me devastated.

But I know deep in my heart that it was the right decision at that time. I made a promise to myself that whenever I started a family it would be with somebody I truly loved and respected, somebody who loved and respected me and wanted to be with me and be there for that child. A relationship that would be for keeps, for ever. That's how I consoled myself – still console myself – when I have moments of regret that I never had that child, that little spirit, that I didn't give them a chance in this life. I hope they have forgiven me, because I have struggled over the years to forgive myself.

Abortion is a difficult subject to talk about openly. It still amazes me that most people will know someone who has had one, but very few will talk about it. I know exactly how it feels and I do wish that people were more accepting and less judgemental of those who, for whatever reason, choose this path.

In the years that followed that experience I became cold and cynical. It was never a choice between my career and a family; in retrospect, I think I was just caught up in the romantic notion of wanting to be in the perfect partnership before starting a family – and also I never found 'The One' until it was too late.

At one point I did consider having a baby on my own as soon as I felt ready. When I heard about the 'Einstein sperm bank' in LA, I joked about it often to friends, but I did think that could be my back-up plan. Brilliantly intelligent sperm (I will bring the looks) would mean I could have the most amazing child and I'd do it all by myself, as I don't need a man. This is still an option for many women, and if it's right for you, then I say go for it. Personally, I never went beyond the initial idea. I think part of the reason is because I feel very blessed; I have five kids around me in my family, so I never feel childless, which helps me tremendously; and I know for a fact that I couldn't love those kids any more if they were my own. But I would also be hiding something if I didn't concede that over the last ten years, seeing my sisters have children has stirred up a mix of feelings and emotions for me. On the one hand, I am overjoyed at being an auntie and at seeing my sisters being loving mums, but I also experience sadness that this won't be happening for me.

Each time my sisters were pregnant I felt a wave of complex emotions; I would be completely overwhelmed with happiness and worry (that they and the babies were going to be OK) in equal measure, tinged with a tiny bit of envy. That isn't a nice emotion to feel when you love someone, and I have always been too ashamed to admit it out loud, so I've just kept it hidden, buried within. You aren't supposed to feel this way about the people you love, are you? I wonder if you can relate to this?

It's possibly the worst feeling to experience, and one you feel you must work hard to hide. Even now, I have a small pang of envy on discovering a friend or someone I know is expecting a baby. It is a perplexing reaction and one that leaves me feeling sad. I would never begrudge anyone starting or extending a family. Quite the opposite – I am genuinely overjoyed. So maybe this feeling is a subconscious maternal longing that sits deep in the fibre of my very being. If I am brutally honest, the envy that I am talking about is not a dangerous green envy; it's more of a sad, melancholy feeling of being left behind, of missing out, feeling lonely or a sense that I have failed at being a woman. The realisation that I will never have that maternal connection with someone who is my own flesh and blood can be hard to accept.

Around the time my niece Willow was born, I went to see my gynaecologist for blood tests to check my AMH (anti-mullarian hormone) levels and see if there might still be a chance for me to have my own baby. I remember the doctor being frustrated with me for asking for these tests and trying to persuade me otherwise, saying she thought the possibility of me being able to conceive were probably very low anyway due to my age. I had just turned forty-one, and thought that as I still felt young and looked younger than my age, everything might still be in perfect working order and my body might cheat the system, so to speak.

I had driven round to see my youngest sister, Jo, and to spend time with Finley and little Willow – something I used to do often, giving her a hand whenever I could because the children were born only eighteen months apart and she welcomed the help. The doctor called to give me the test results, and I knew from her cold, neutral tone as soon as I answered the phone that the news she was about to give me was exactly as she had expected and that my levels were so low that I was unlikely to ever be able to have a baby. There were no kind words offered – just a bold, frank statement devoid of any emotion.

At that moment I felt as if I had been punched in the stomach, and as I held my newborn niece in my arms, tears rolled down my face, my heart broken. I was furious and angry, not only at the way the doctor had delivered the news, but also at my life and my situation. It felt so cruel, and I couldn't make any sense of it. I just couldn't believe that after all these years of being on the pill, of trying each month to NOT get pregnant while I was with some loser boyfriend, my body was now saying, nope, it's not possible, you can't, it's too late. I stayed the night with my sister, and drank a bottle of wine, quickly, to numb the pain.

Was this my fault? Was it a punishment? After all, I had had my chance to have a baby and I had chosen not to, hadn't I? Maybe you don't get many chances. Maybe I had made a very wrong decision almost twenty years before, and now it was too late.

Or was it?

Not satisfied with the no and the brush-off from the gynaecologist, I decided to go and see a specialist to enquire about freezing my eggs. Once again, there were blood tests and a more in-depth investigation. This time, it was a kinder experience. The doctor was gentle as he explained that I had a very slim chance of being able to have a baby that way. The retrieval process is tricky in itself. The doctors checked my ovaries to see how many follicles they were producing, which would give them an idea of how many eggs could be retrieved. Even though I did have a few follicles, the quality of the eggs he might retrieve, again due to my age (goddamn it, why hadn't I looked into this years before?) would probably not survive the thawing process. I would have had a better chance if I had a partner and we could potentially have frozen the embryo. Well, I didn't have a partner, so that was that. He said I might have a slight chance of conceiving naturally, but that it was very slim. When I asked what that chance would be, he replied that it was 3 per cent. Not the best odds, really. Again, I was crestfallen.

So, I parked the baby thing and concentrated on my career, working hard, and somehow continuing to date inappropriate, emotionally unavailable men. Some six to eight months later, I was in a relationship – albeit a rather destructive one. Early one morning, as I was getting ready to leave for my breakfast radio show, I drank a glass of juice and immediately had to run to the bathroom, vomiting violently. And, just like the first time, I felt, almost instinctively, that I might be pregnant. As unbelievable as I thought it could be, it had to be morning sickness – something I had never experienced in my life before. I went to work and tried not to get too excited, keeping it all to myself.

This time, even though the relationship wasn't perfect, I saw it as a sign from the universe – maybe from God – that I had been forgiven and I was finally going to have a baby. I was going to be a mum. I am not religious, but it was hard not to feel blessed at that moment, given the odds. I felt reprieved.

I got through the show and picked up some tests on my way home. And, sure enough, I was pregnant. WOW! There I was, defying all odds, after all the doctors, the tests, the no, it's too late. I knew it, I knew it – my body was still fertile and I should never have worried.

There was no doubt that I would keep this baby. The relationship wasn't ideal, far from it, but I felt I was being given a chance again and I was happy about it. Of course, it wasn't as straightforward as all that, though. Over the next eight weeks I had weekly scans to monitor my progress due to my age. The scans showed that the baby wasn't growing as it should, and the heartbeat was very faint, which deeply concerned the doctors, who were trying their best to manage my expectations at every appointment. I tried to keep calm, happy and positive during those early weeks and months, although it was a very stressful time. Again, going to scans and appointments alone was not ideal, but I was older, and I could handle it better.

Then, one morning when I was at work, I started bleeding. I rushed to the bathroom, full of panic at seeing all that blood. I didn't know what to do. We'd only just gone on air, and I knew I had to keep working. I dug deep and tried to park the dread I felt in the pit of my stomach, praying that my baby would be OK. As soon as the show was finished and we were off air, I rushed to the hospital. I still don't know how I did that show, with all the worry and concern, my head spinning. When I arrived, my worst fears were confirmed – the scan showed that the heartbeat had stopped. My baby had died.

To say I was devastated was an understatement; I was heartbroken, inconsolable. My amazing friend Caroline met me there. I'd called her after the show in tears, explaining what was happening as I rushed to the hospital. She held my hand and sobbed with me while the doctor did the scans and delivered the sad news. I will never forget how she felt my pain as if she was experiencing it herself, it made my heart break even more.

I have since done so much work to heal and let go of the idea of being a mum, but I still remember this moment so clearly and am still choked up writing about it now. I am convinced the reason for my miscarriage was yes, partly due to the egg quality, but also because my partner had attacked me in the street the night before, shaking me violently and throwing me up against some metal shop-front shutters.

That was my rock bottom, the moment of realisation that I needed to change my life, change what I thought about myself, to get some sense of self-worth and stop making the same mistakes. It was time I grew up.

It was becoming clear that, for whatever reason, I wasn't meant to be a mum. I think I have had too much healing to do in other areas of my life and, who knows, if we do come back in another life, maybe I will be more evolved and ready to be a parent. I didn't want to be in a state of self-pity, but I had to be realistic and think of the bigger picture – I could be there as a mother figure for my sisters, to look after my mum and dad, and I know I am an epic auntie to those little cuties I love so much. I am also a realist and know this is a part of life and natural selection and that the baby might have had something seriously wrong with it. Sometimes nature takes over, and that's what has helped me come to terms with it.

I am what I call a 'work in progress'; I have a few wobbles every now and again, moments of melancholy and of what could have been, but over the years, this feeling has lessened and now it doesn't consume my every thought. Thank goodness, as I would find that very hard to live with.

To come to terms with it, I have had to reframe what my life looks like now and what my future looks like, to see how blessed I am, regardless, rather than wishing for what I can't have or what can no longer be. This tactic makes it possible for me to compartmentalise aspects of my life and enables me to be realistic and move on without more heartache and disappointment. This has become easier as time has passed, but for many years it wasn't so easy. When your only ambition growing up is to become a mum, it takes some serious recalibrating and reconfiguring in your head, maybe some therapy, too, to change that destiny in your mind. But as we know, time is a healer.

Although I have somehow put to bed the pain of a life without children, that is not to say I don't adore them and find them compelling to watch. Seeing them working things out, their joy and curiosity, their eyes sparkling with mischief and wonder. I also appreciate that staring at other people's kids is not an appropriate thing to do or to admit to, and it must look a little strange sometimes! I do check myself (or George does it for me), as I'm fascinated by watching families, looking out for mannerisms and certain behaviours, or seeing how DNA has passed between them. I will notice the child's curls from their mum or brown eyes from their dad, different skin tones and beautiful cultures combined. I daydream about what my child might have looked like.

The laughter and wonder of kids bring me so much joy. Whenever I see babies, I want to cuddle or hold them – that maternal instinct always there, bubbling beneath the surface. When I see pregnant women, I feel happy for them, and the miracle of birth always leaves me in tears, completely overcome with emotion and amazement at the wonder of life.

For my part, I console myself knowing that I have a wonderful life – maybe not the one I thought was going to be mine – and I remind myself of that as often as I can. I am happy with my life as it is – George and me, just the two of us – and I relish what we have. Living with this attitude is so much kinder than craving or pining for something I can't have. I have had to become mentally strong to move on, my logical brain having to override a lot of the feelings when they surface. My main priority is that I want to be happy. I don't want to live with regret or have a huge cloud hanging over me, constantly living with sadness.

This is such a huge topic, and I could write about so many different aspects of it, but if you have a friend who has never had children, I do hope this gives a small insight into how they might be feeling as they reach menopause. There are so many things that happen in the life of a woman and reaching perimenopause can feel like the point of no return. It is scary, regardless of whether you have children or not.

If you have struggled with fertility, I am so sorry. I appreciate that I am one of the luckier ones because I have made peace with it, and I want to offer my sympathies to you if, after trying for many years, it hasn't happened for you, or if you have lost a child or a baby and your heart is irreparably broken. I am deeply sorry, I truly am. I do believe talking can really help; speaking to a grief counsellor or a therapist can offer comfort to work through the pain, the heartache, the sadness and the disappointment.

I have friends who have tried every avenue to have a baby. They haven't taken no for an answer, and I respect that; they are stronger than me. I saw not having a baby more as a sign that for me it wasn't meant to be, and I also saw how relationships get tested during the heartbreaking process of trying every treatment available, so I decided it wasn't for me. Egg donors, sperm donors, IVF, adoption – the pressure can sometimes be too much for a couple. It's an all-consuming and expensive process. Some people go as far as remortgaging their homes, not to mention putting their bodies through so much with all the hormone therapy and more. In desperation, many people just throw money at the situation, and there is a lot of money to be made from couples who are going through fertility issues. (I see this with some expensive menopause doctors out there, too, preying on women who are vulnerable and will do anything just to feel better.)

When George and I first got back together it was not long after my miscarriage and I had left my unhappy relationship. I was honest with him, explaining everything I had been through and what I had learned about my fertility situation. We had this beautiful, open conversation where he expressed how grateful he was that we had found one another again after all these years, and that if it was just the two of us, that would be all he needed. It immediately took the pressure off, and I felt immense gratitude to him for such a grown-up, mature and brilliant attitude. George eased the situation, and made me see it from a different point of view. I wanted to continue talking about it, but I was thrilled at his initial reaction and it changed and shifted something in me, too. I felt my shoulders relax, as all the heaviness I had put on myself – the burden of explaining my fertility challenge and the shame I felt – left my body.

I was still getting pressure from certain friends, though, who, knowing I was finally in a healthy, solid relationship, wanted me to see their amazing doctors or specialists so that I could have it all, with a baby to boot. I think I got caught up in that vision and their enthusiasm, so I decided to give it one last shot. I got the name of a supposedly incredible fertility doctor who had helped a friend of mine through IVF for both her babies, and who also came highly recommended through another friend. This time George came with me to the appointment, knowing that it was something I wanted to explore. Being the intelligent, logical man he is, he of course asked all the right questions, challenged the doctor and explained everything I had been through. It turned out that the success rate couldn't be confirmed but it wasn't likely to be that high, and it would also be a very expensive process to even begin to try. I walked out of the appointment feeling somewhat confused – slightly hopeful, possibly deluded.

George brought me straight back down to earth with a bang. We went out for dinner, ordered a bottle of wine and threw it all out on the table, deciding that the two of us were all we needed, that our love was strong enough and that we would have a life full of fun and adventures instead of having a child. And that was when I realised I was going to be OK not being a mum. I still had moments of hope, though, that maybe, just maybe, I might be surprised one month and we might conceive – that old, unshakeable, maternal instinct still hanging around in the background.

It floors me now to think back to the constant pressure from (mostly female) editors and journalists to explain why I hadn't had a baby or why I wasn't trying to conceive. I had to endure their judgement and that of others in the press, as they assumed I was so ambitious and career-driven, so selfish, that having a baby wasn't on my to-do list. It even worked against me professionally at times; I remember a top TV executive explaining to me that the reason I didn't get a primetime music show was because I wasn't a mother and nor was I married, which made me a threat to certain viewers. They believed that people watching – in particular women – wouldn't 'get' me, as I hadn't gone down the traditional route.

Thankfully, times are changing (not quickly enough, if you ask me), but that doesn't alter how it has been for those of us ladies who either chose not to have children or have found it hard to do so.

Not everyone can conceive at the drop of a hat; not everyone is in a situation that allows children to happen. There are so many variables, unique to each of us. More sensitivity and less judgement are needed around this subject, as everyone's journey is different. Some people's lack of tact or delicacy baffles me. And it also blows me away that well into my mid-forties, and even now sometimes, people offer up suggestions and advice on how I could still be a mum, as if I have never considered all the options. It used to make me so sad that no one really knew what I had been through physically or mentally.

I also want to say that more women need to be honest about how children impact their lives. Yes, of course this happens in the most positive way, because they are joyful and beautiful and, hopefully, born out of love – if you love your partner, a child can be the natural next step. But women also need to come out and be brutally honest about their situations – because as cute as they are, kids can be ungrateful little gits, what with the sleepless nights, the endless demands, the cost, how much it drains you, etc. Kids are just the best thing in the world, but there's also a flip side, where it's bloody hard work and really is a struggle sometimes, and you spend so many years putting yourself ever-lower down on that growing list of priorities. Sometimes it's just good to be super honest about how hard parenting is as well. I hear from so many perimenopausal and menopausal women who find it hell on earth to be not only dealing with their hormones raging out of control, but also living with and raising teenagers who are experiencing drastic changes in their own bodies, too. The guilt that comes from the clashing generations and explosive outbursts from both parties, leaves them drained and exhausted and wracked with guilt. I take my hat off to you women who somehow manage to do it all, finding time to raise a family, hold down a career and run a house. A friend of mine who shall remain anonymous once said about his kids that it's the most fun you'll ever have being miserable!

Still, there's always that little, tiny thought in my head and in my heart about what having a baby with George would be like. I see him with my nieces and nephews, and he's such an amazing uncle. I can only imagine how fantastic he would have been as a dad. I think he's so smart and loving, and kind and nurturing, and it would melt my heart into a million trillion pieces to see him like that. But that wasn't meant for us.

We could have gone down the adoption road, although when we got back together it was getting a little late and the process is really long. Although I am moved by babies and the miracle of birth, I don't regret the decision we made to just be together and have our beautiful life. We go on many adventures, loving each other to our full capacity. When I tell friends what we are doing on a weekend or about a trip we have planned, some of them exclaim, 'Oh, I am so envious of your life!' or, 'You have so many great adventures together. You can do so many things.' And it's true. If we want to stay in bed on a Saturday morning watching documentaries, that's what we do. Some weekends, not all – as we're usually early risers – we can sit in bed in the morning with a fresh pot of coffee enjoying time that's just for us. I do have more time for myself; some people might see me as selfish, but this is the life that happened for me and, in a way, I guess this is the life I chose.

Life is challenging enough, work is challenging enough, and for us to have added a baby into the mix when I was in my mid-forties would have been absolute crazy town. I would have been perimenopausal as well, so maybe not the best mother I could have been. I mean, it's horrible to say that and obviously I would have dug deep, and I would have had plenty of support, but I just don't think I would have been able to cope.

So I think sometimes the universe gives you what's meant for you. It gives you what you can handle, what you can cope with, and I truly believe that life goes full circle and you start to become responsible for the people who were responsible for you. My mum will call me a nag because I'm always telling her what she should be doing and what food she should be eating. I'll send my dad collagen supplements and probiotics for his stomach, and for his general wellbeing I'll send him all sorts of vitamins and minerals. He's so well behaved these days; he always takes them (or at least he tells me that he does). And I enjoy all this – the sense of responsibility comforts me, because I do love to nurture and look after people.

In the past, I put other people before myself. In fact, I did so for years and years. But recently, I have started to redress this balance. I've always said in my social media Self-care Sundays (and about self-care in general) that you can't give from an empty cup, which basically means you have to conserve your energy and be well in yourself in order to be present and able to take care of others around you. And you can only do that if you truly put yourself at the top of the list.

Finally, I believe that my life so far has been a journey of growth and learning. My time here was meant for me to work on myself, to be tested and challenged. I love my life, I really do. I have come to see that life is beautiful and challenging, and it is hard to make plans because everything changes. Life changes. So, there is no point in wondering what could have been.

I am a firm believer that there is still so much for me to learn. In life you can either dwell on the past and long for something different or put on your big-girl pants, see life as a glass half full and appreciate your situation, despite the disappointment of not being entirely satisfied.

LIFE GOES ON

I have changed massively as a person throughout my life – even just in the last few years. What I now know that I deserve and want in my life, as opposed to what I do not want, is so clear-cut, and the universe knows that, too, and conspires to give me what I want. And it will do the same for you, too. The longing for youth, the mourning of a life passing too fast, and self-loathing and dark depression can

all be things of the past. I have a very onwards-and-up-
wards attitude now. I try to seek out a higher vibration
through my meditative work, and I strive to achieve a
higher, more satisfying sense of self. I am mindful of not
staying stuck in the past and what was.

There are many life hacks and mental adjustments that
can help us to learn to love ourselves – like cranking up the
self-care, nurturing our minds, unravelling past trauma
and hurt, breaking old patterns and habits that cause us to
have negative, unhealthy thoughts of self-hatred and relationships to break down. Once we learn new techniques,
laugh a lot more, talk more, share what is happening to us
and how we feel (after all, sharing is caring), we will start
to feel more positive, notice when the negative voice pops
up and be able to crush it just as quickly.

What breaks my heart is for far too long women have
just dealt with this all alone – with the confusion, the pain
and the struggle. It's been swept under the carpet, amid
feelings of shame and embarrassment, with people being
too afraid to admit or share experiences and consequently
suffering in silence. This is just not acceptable any more.

I have already shared what I know about the symptoms
of the perimenopause and the menopause and how these
can trigger outbursts of anger, rage, depression, sadness,
loneliness, sleep deprivation, anxiety, dark moods, hot
flushes, lack of libido and the general feeling that you are
losing your mind. In the next part, I will share how I expe-

rienced these changes and how I came to deal with them. I don't want you to feel that you don't understand what is happening to you and you have nowhere to turn.

Getting through the menopause starts with changing our attitude: we need to be pro-ageing, and incorporate mindfulness, movement and good nutrition into our life-styles, as well as understand the benefits of HRT. And we need to be able to talk it all through with no judgement and a lot of patience. So, let's keep going!

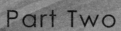

Part Two

Eye of the Storm

If you would have told me ten years ago that as a 51-year-old woman I would be fully into my menopause, post-menopause even, I would never have believed you. After all, it was only seven, eight years ago that I was considering the possibility of having a baby!

The image of a menopausal woman in my mind did not look like me, and certainly didn't act like me, and I think that is true for so many of us women. I believed it was something that happened when we got much older, like much, much older. Society has always shunned the older woman, especially in the Western world, seeing them as no longer of childbearing age, no longer relevant in society, no longer desirable, basically washed up, forgotten. Getting older is, of course, going to happen to us all, but feeling and looking our age is not going to be an option, not on my watch. I still want to wear my hair in plaits and put on an oversized pair of dungarees from time to time, wear all the colours and clash my prints, and I will continue to do this, wearing what I want for ever. This idea of dressing 'age appropriately' really gets my back up. My advice? Wear whatever the fuck you want, sister!

The ageist attitude sickens me to my stomach; it makes me angry and breaks my heart to think of the women who have gone before me, struggling alone, too afraid to express how they were feeling, scared, their health deteriorating – almost crumbling before their eyes – because they were no longer deemed important. The fact is, we are now living longer than ever before, which means we all need help, support and advice even more, as well as understanding in all areas of our lives. We can do so much to help ourselves look and feel fantastic, in both our minds and bodies. Diet and exercise are crucial – I cannot stress this enough – as they are the path to a healthier, happier you, making you stronger, both mentally and physically, and more in control, with improved sleep as well as confidence.

So, let's get started.

CONFRONTING NEGATIVITY

I am healthy, and as I have mentioned before, I have made some huge changes in my life since I entered perimenopause. I see my health as a 360-degree approach that I must take full responsibility for. I know what I need to do to help myself daily, to heal myself and how I need to live my life.

I have a sense of self-acceptance knowing that I am older, that I am not the same girl I was in my twenties. Nor do I want to be – I like who I am now, even with some of the war wounds I carry, and I am living my best menopausal life. It is great, I promise, once you are through some of the trickier times and you are looking after yourself.

But before we can shed the negativity and start to heal, we need to deal with what was in the past. There are many things that may have happened to all of us that perhaps weren't addressed at the time. Some people don't even appear to register when something goes wrong and it goes completely unrecorded, as if nothing has happened.

However, no matter how much we consciously or unconsciously repress and bury issues, events and specific moments over the years, we still carry the bruises and imperceptible scars that cause us pain. Sometimes thoughts float across my mind – unanswered questions, such as, is this all there is? I wonder if something is missing? Or I get that feeling that I have either lost something or been left behind. Should I feel more content? Could I be happier? The disappointments of my past, some of the unresolved pain and frustration, keep me from fulfilling and living my true potential and it drags me down. And I know I want these feelings to be gone for good.

I have been working on myself while writing this book. I was doing really well, and it was cathartic to write all these words and set down what I have been through. I thought I had it sorted, and life was good. However, we travelled to Japan, where I decided to have a digital detox, which meant no phone time at all. This was a first for me.

I was content to exercise each day, sometimes walking as many as 20,000 steps while taking in Tokyo life and looking up at the wondrous architecture. My little note-book was always in my bag in case I had any ideas to write down. The strange quietness, the respite from the social media world I had been living in, gave me an immense sense of mental clarity. It engulfed me, and then I felt an odd, heavy, physical pain in my shoulder. In that instant, I knew what that pain was.

It was an old injury that has plagued me for the last thirty-two years. Except it was no ordinary injury. I didn't slip on a wet floor or pull a muscle playing tennis. I am sad to admit, that it was the result of domestic abuse at the hands of a bully I unfortunately dated for too many years.

Like so many cases of domestic abuse, it started as mental abuse, the man in question controlling me through what I now know was clearly gaslighting – a term that we have come to understand only recently. Well, this happened to me for very many years. I was in my late teens and he was older than me, although I didn't know this at the time, as he had lied to me about his age. The physical abuse came soon after the mental abuse.

He was a man about town, pretty popular, so imagine my surprise when he was interested in me! Because I was young, my self-worth had not yet developed and, coming from a broken home, I had that sense of sadness already setting in. With all my deep-rooted insecurities flashing like a beacon for all to see, he latched on, and things got progressively worse.

Now, remember I was used to being bullied at school, so initially I didn't register his words as evil, or his nastiness and disrespectful attitude towards me. I just accepted the situation. Yes, of course it hurt me, and I have come to realise that words cut so much deeper than physical abuse, their impact creating such a blow that I don't think you can ever forget them.

This is how it started: words, digs, taking advantage of me, chipping away more and more at my self-confidence and my self-esteem. Bullying behaviour, pure and simple. I had just been asked by a model scout if I was interested in becoming a model; this was not something that had ever crossed my mind, as I never considered myself good looking or attractive enough. In my mind, Christy Turlington and Linda Evangelista were models. But me? Just a skinny little thing from Welwyn Garden City. Anyway, after a few weeks thinking about it I decided, why not, let's see what this modelling agency was offering.

And thank goodness I did, as that decision changed my life. I stayed with the small, independent agency for a year, and while I was working with a very respectable photographer, he suggested I change to a bigger, more established agency. At this point, my relationship started to deteriorate further. His temper got worse, as he picked on me constantly, and not content with using all my money (he didn't make any at all), he also cheated on me repeatedly while I was off on shoots. I know now he was deeply insecure and, in turn, tried to make me feel that way to keep control and power, which of course worked, as I wasn't into mind games and certainly didn't understand that was what was going on. I found out finally about one cheating incident as he gave me a very nasty STD – the kind that only comes from putting it about, a lot. I was mortified. Nineteen years old and riddled with a vile sexually transmitted infection. It made my blood boil, and I felt beyond disgusted.

His words were getting more and more evil, his controlling nature more sinister. I will never know why I stayed as long as I did, I guess I thought that was love and that people argued and maybe I deserved to be bullied and picked on. I didn't know that the worst was yet to come.

He started to use physical violence against me. When I threatened to leave, he would hold me up against a wall, both of his hands around my throat, my feet dangling off the ground and squeeze my neck and strangle me until I thought I would die. This happened so many times I lost count. I never told a soul.

Emotionally, I was broken. I felt unworthy of love, but he would also be so upset after all his angry violent outbursts, and so full of remorse, that I would have to comfort him and tell him it was going to be OK. I mean, how fucked up is that?

One time, he was chasing me and kicking me, and to protect myself from another of his kicks I used my arm to cover my backside. He kicked my arm with all his power, and I heard a crack. Sure enough, the damage had been done and my arm was in plaster for six weeks or so. The position of my arm being twisted around my back and broken caused me, and still causes me, so much pain. Over the years, I developed a condition called scoliosis (curvature of the spine), which can occur after an impact trauma. In my case, my left shoulder and scapula now pull forwards as a result of the injury, thus curving my spine to the left. He also headbutted me one day, knocking me unconscious, clean out, leaving me with a huge black eye. How I didn't die in the flat, I will never know.

As I write this, I still feel such a huge sense of anger at how anyone could do that to a young girl. I am in tears, but I mostly feel sad, for my younger self – so lost, scared and alone.

Remember, I was working as a model in those days, and would turn up to work, arm in plaster, with bruises and a black eye, having to come up with the most elaborate excuses to protect him. I have had to work so hard on my feelings of forgiveness, and truthfully it has not been easy.

Admitting this to you now, I hope it may save the life of someone who is the victim of an abuser. If any of my family, my young and innocent nieces or nephews, ever experienced this kind of evil, I don't think I could be held responsible for what I would do to their abuser. I know that's not really what I should be saying, but I still have a lot of anger inside me, and I guess some regret. It has been years, and I mean years, of sadness, reflection and confusion as to why it happened to me, and how I allowed it, how I found it acceptable.

So, going back to the Japan trip. Being off my phone, off social media and having no distractions meant that I was aware of the pain being so intense that it made even walking painful. I have had numerous shiatsu treatments to try to help with the agony, and I follow a daily gym session involving lots of stretching. I have also been opening up more to George about the feelings and sensations coming up from this injury, one of which I have never spoken about before – the intense pain along my spine and into my shoulder and neck, which brings back the pain and anger I hold deep within the very fibre of my being. I have had to work hard to forgive a man who hurt me so badly and left lasting scars, both physical and emotional, that I have to live with. And yet, I now come at this from a place of understanding, as I have learned that to hurt someone you must have been deeply hurt yourself, so he was acting from pain himself, and maybe he has never dealt with it.

That is how I have to view it in order to forgive and move on – although, admittedly, some days this is easier said than done.

FORGIVENESS

Forgiveness starts with you, with me, with us. We must make a conscious decision to let go of the things that are bothering and distressing us; we need to work through whatever has happened to us, to enable us to move forwards with our lives.

To do this, first we must forgive ourselves – for the guilt over situations we might have found ourselves in over the years, for the lies we told to protect ourselves or someone else while we were in the thick of it, for the shame we feel about having let ourselves get into a situation – as well as the people who caused us that harm.

I admit that releasing feelings of anger and resentment is not always easy. It takes time and work – and it can take years. Be patient, though, because I promise it will be worth it.

I see forgiveness as not dissimilar to self-acceptance. It is easier to love than to hate, and to live with forgiveness puts so much less pressure on us, making us feel lighter in body, mind and soul. Without feelings of bitterness, we can breathe more easily and sleep more soundly. What I know from experience is that living with a constant sense of anger and resentment towards people who have wronged us is a total waste of energy. Harbouring that anger is not healthy; repressing those emotions and burying them deep inside not only prevents us from moving on and from attracting what we rightly deserve in our lives, but it also dulls our sparkle, stops us from vibrating at our highest level and closes us off to incredible possibilities. Instead of using that precious energy on hating, we could be channelling it so much more positively and using it in a more constructive way to enrich our lives.

While forgiveness is so important, I will say that you don't ever forget. Those wounds, whether mental or physical, take a long time to heal. And maybe they don't ever entirely heal; perhaps they leave scars that stay with you. But you will learn to live with those scars and realise that they make you who you are. That they are a part of what makes you *you*.

Whatever happened happened, and from time to time that trauma may rear its ugly head, but I have learned how to manage my emotions on those occasions. I will have a cry to release the tension and the sadness, or I might scream, or go for a long walk, or throw myself into an exercise class or a run.

Sometimes, we don't know our own strength and how what we can overcome is incredible – we are so much more resilient than we realise and we must always give ourselves credit for this. It is important that we acknowledge how far we have come from whatever uncomfortable situation we have been in, and that way we can truly appreciate what we have now. Having said that, we are all human, and some days are easier than others. But for me, realising that I am who I am because of those wounds and scars gives me comfort and reminds me that I am courageous, I am fierce, I am a fighter – and so are you.

To feel extreme gratitude and happiness for the life I have now brings me such a warm feeling of comfort and security. I know that whoever hurt me in the past can't hurt me ever again. I survived – well, actually, I chose to thrive – and I want you to do the same.

I have had trips away by myself to reflect on my life over the years, to come to terms with and understand that the situations I've come up against are maybe lessons. To feel more empathy than anger towards the person or people that have caused you harm is truly a liberating and empowering way to ease the heavy burden of hurt.

Therapy has helped me – not only talking to a counsellor, but many other alternative treatments, which I will continue to try more of because I feel that the power of touch from healers and therapists – whoever helps with mind or body – brings me huge amounts of comfort. I saw a shaman years ago after a bad break-up, when all the hurt and betrayal rolled into one, and together we performed ceremonies to help heal and let go of the sadness, disappointment and hurt I felt. I have done regression therapy, too, where I screamed so loud and felt my whole body shaking with so much rage and anger that I thought I might combust. The feeling was so intense; I had no idea I could feel like that, and the therapist who I worked with was visibly shaken – he also felt what I was feeling as he led me through this process. It was mind-blowing, extremely revealing and completely inexplicable, but it helped me to move through this pent-up anger and resentment.

Other therapies I have tried include hypnotherapy, deep body treatments and craniosacral therapy, which is incredible. The therapist barely touches you, but you feel the flow of sacral fluids moving in and around the nervous system to help alleviate pain. It is fantastic for all-over health and immunity. I sought comfort with this treatment after I broke up with the bully, as I felt it helped my body to eliminate some of the pain it had been holding on to. I would be in tears as I lay there, a sense of relief washing over me, and when her hands travelled up towards my throat, hovering over that area, I would always have a panic attack, my body reminding me of the repetitive trauma that area had suffered. It was a very nurturing way to heal after five years of abuse. Craniosacral therapy is also ideal if you aren't ready to discuss anything with a therapist just yet. Reiki healing is another beautiful and gentle treatment, where the therapist uses energy healing to help move through the body and unblock and free areas of stagnation within the body caused by repressed emotions or trauma. I would recommend both, although I would also say that you have to be open to them and have an element of trust.

I wasn't brave enough to ask for help. I also thought that it was a sign of weakness to go to therapy. But I now understand that we must show up for ourselves and do what we need to do to forgive ourselves and others and move on. Please don't see it as weakness, because true weakness is when you do not deal with your pain and then get ill years later because you bottled it all up.

If you prefer to keep things to yourself, writing things down and journaling is so good for getting your thoughts out; or if talking face to face is more your thing, share your thoughts with your friends – it is such a good way to get things out of your system and process them, so you can move on more easily.

This is how I have worked on forgiveness and healing. I now feel sorry for all the people who have hurt me. I see them as sad, lonely and very damaged – because to inflict pain and suffering on another human being (or any living thing) is a very sad and destructive thing to do, and I am sure that makes them very unhappy. I have come to understand that often the abuser has been abused themselves or has witnessed abuse as a child within a family dynamic. Knowing this helps me to forgive, if not forget, so that I can put the past hurts to bed and enjoy the life I now have.

FINDING POSITIVITY AND SUPPORT

Looking back, my first symptoms of perimenopause started not long after I lost the baby in my early forties. I was overcome with anxiety, stress and felt completely over-emotional.

Now some of you will say I had plenty of reason for that – and I did. There had been the miscarriage, we had also lost our beloved Nanna Nora, so I guess I was experiencing a heavy combination of grief and the hormones from the pregnancy. Added to that, I had been in a very turbulent relationship.

I threw myself into intense weekly therapy sessions with a counsellor, as well as cognitive behavioural therapy (CBT) to reset and retrain my brain into changing the way I reacted to things. As part of this, I learned to look at the patterns that had formed since my childhood, to discuss and work out why I was at rock bottom again, and in a similar situation with abusive relationships – why I was continually making the same mistakes with men, attracting the wrong kind and, in turn, hurting myself.

On the suggestion of the counsellor, I took a year off from relationships and refrained from texting men or flirting with them; I had absolutely no dates at all, basically doing a dating detox to understand what I truly wanted from life and from a partner, and working to get in touch and reconnect with myself.

I know that I had mostly jumped into relationships far too quickly and without listening to my gut instinct or intuition on whether they were what I wanted, whether we were suited or if they were good for me (this last point is the most important one).

I took that time to really work out where I had been going wrong, where I had done myself a disservice by not following that intuition, ignoring the warning signs that were always so apparent and blatantly disregarding the red flags. This, I knew, needed to stop, if I was to have any happiness, and a peaceful, loving relationship.

Throughout that year, I did, however, connect with one man. We went to bed together every night, with me always falling asleep to his wise words sinking into my subconscious.

That man was Deepak Chopra.

I had been aware of his teachings, but had never used them to really focus on manifesting what I wanted for my future. I listened on my phone to the music, the power of his words, over and over each night. I didn't always completely understand everything and usually fell asleep somewhere during the *The Secret of Healing: Meditations for Transformation and Higher Consciousness* (I still listen to this from time to time and have recommended it to countless friends), but around two months in, I started to feel a lightness – almost a connection to my higher self – and I was calmer, more grounded. I wasn't missing having dates or dinners with men, nor was I interested in any pointless casual flirtations. I now saw that validation I had always sought out – to lift me, to confirm that I was desirable, attractive, who knows? – for what it was: a pathetic boost to my ego, and an instant gratification that was short-lived and completely unnecessary.

It seemed ridiculous that I had used validation from strangers to fill a hole of self-doubt and self-worth. No wonder I was so quick to let narcissistic people in. I could see more clearly where I had been on a loop, constantly repeating the same mistakes, using alcohol and sex to fill a void of something huge that was missing: my sense of true self-worth and self-love. You can never truly love another if you don't have love and respect for yourself. Love starts with yourself.

I felt I had hit rock bottom so many times and I knew I needed to make changes. The power was in my hands, and it was all down to me to break this repetitive streak of self-destruction. This was when I introduced manifestation into my life. Each evening, I would lie in bed, looking up, and write an imaginary list on the ceiling of what I wanted from a partner and a relationship. Then, before I turned on Deepak, I would breathe deeply and again list out all the qualities I knew to be important in my future life partner, my teammate, my lover, my best friend, throwing it out to the universe:

- Kind
- Loving
- Good work ethic
- Handsome
- Tall
- To have a beautiful relationship with his mum
- Ambitious
- Funny
- Find me funny
- A sense of adventure

Each night I added to this, as more qualities I knew to be important to me would reveal themselves. The list grew long, and my heart started to feel full. I felt excited. I could almost feel this person already in my life. I practised this for months and months: early nights, staying in, cooking for myself, making my manifestation list on the ceiling, drifting off to sleep, listening to my beloved Deepak all the while. The list continued to grow, as there were elements I realised I had left out, and I didn't want to omit a single crucial thing.

Around eight months later, I received a phone call from a dear friend of mine.

The conversation went something like this.

ME: Hi my love, how are you?

AMANDA: Lis! How you doing?

ME: I am good, honey. I am just on my way to switch on the Oxford Street Christmas lights.

AMANDA: OK. Listen, Lis, so there is this guy that you used to date—

And I swear to God in that moment I knew I could finish her sentence. It came to me in a flash, a person and a name, someone I hadn't seen or thought of for years. I said:

ME: Wait, is his name George Smart?

AMANDA: Yes! How the hell did you know?

ME: Honestly, I have no idea. I just knew it. His name just came to me as you were talking.

Spooky? Yes! Coincidental? Not really. I know now that the universe conspires to give you what you want when you send out your wishes, dreams and intentions – that certainty of what you want for your life. Now I didn't realise then that I had manifested George to come back into my life at a time when I was ready and clear that he was the man I had been searching for. He was the guy on my invisible ceiling list.

George Smart is a man I'd met almost fifteen years before in our MTV days. I was a VJ on air and he had come fresh from uni and was head of all their big events – basically putting together shows with Trevor Nelson and Russell Brand. We ended up kissing in a field at the V Festival one year, after working through the weekend interviewing bands and acts for the show. He is seven years younger than me, and with me being almost thirty at the time that seemed like the biggest and most ridiculous age gap. I wasn't really into younger men, and I was about to go off to the States to work on a big BBC show, so getting involved with anyone wasn't really on the cards. We ended up having a few dates here and there, and in my eyes it was nothing serious. I didn't think he would be interested in me either, being all those years older, but little did I know that he had always had a crush on me. Anyway, it ended as soon as it started and we went our separate ways, with just a phone call occasionally and him sending me a few messages on Facebook to which I didn't really respond.

The rest is beautiful, romantic history. Amanda gave him my number, he called me and we arranged a date – or, when I say we arranged the date, George did everything! I had been used to having to book restaurants, plan things, but he took over, and even when I told him what kind of food I liked as well as restaurant suggestions he just said, 'Leave it with me'.

I felt completely out of my depth, as well as out of control, not knowing where we were going, and I wondered if we would get on and, most importantly, would I fancy him? It had been so long, and I couldn't find a photo of him anywhere – not on any social platforms and his Facebook account was long gone.

But I jumped in with a leap of faith – and I am glad I did. On the night of the date, the nerves were intense; George had booked Pollen Street Social, a Jason Atherton restaurant just off Hanover Square. I got there a little early, busying myself at the cashpoint machine to waste a few minutes, and then I set off down the tiny street, unsure of what I was doing, as not only had it been a long time since I had been on a date, it had also been fifteen years since George and I had seen one another. Now, unbeknown to me, you can get to the restaurant from two streets, and as I walked down Pollen Street, George was walking up. As we approached each other, we started to smile. It was the same George, only different – he was older, seemed taller, so much more mature. He was a man. Both of us broke into giggles, we hugged and it felt somehow familiar. It was magical.

We didn't stop talking all night, first at the bar, drinking cocktails, then we moved on to the tasting menu. I didn't want the night to end. It was perfect. However, what wasn't perfect was that I had just started on the antidepressants the doctor had prescribed me, and after drinking a mixture of martinis and wine, I felt a little worse for wear.

I have never felt worse in my life than I did the next day. Googling the medication I was taking, I noticed it was advised not to drink. Whoops. I felt like death – but I was so excited about George. After that night, we had a magical week of different dates – again, all organised by George – and since then we haven't left each other's sides.

Since then, he has been my rock, my teammate, my partner – he is my soulmate. He has helped me through some very scary times, and he persevered when I told him I didn't want to be in a relationship, deliberately trying to sabotage what we had as my self-destruct mode tried to kick in because I felt I wasn't worthy of love. I also felt I was too afraid to commit in case I got hurt – that constant reminder that relationships aren't for ever, that they break down and someone is always left heart-broken (and I didn't want that to be me). I hated the vulnerability that comes with giving your heart over to someone, and trusting, really trusting, wasn't something I had ever done before.

George is for keeps – I know that now; but I didn't really know it then. We have been through some serious ups and downs, and he has stood by me, and I him. And he is everything I manifested on my list.

What I want you to take from this is that it can happen to you. You can write the list in your journal or on pieces of paper; don't leave anything out and keep adding to it, going through it and rereading it every day, until you are 100 per cent clear on what you want. Then, when you are ready – or rather, when the universe feels you are ready, because you have done the work and you have love and respect for yourself – it will happen for you. Visualise it, feel it, trust it.

MANAGING ANXIETY

So, I got my rock and my happy ever after. But little did I know that my hormones had another chapter in store for me, another little ride on the rollercoaster. Poor George.

Another thing about perimenopause and menopause is that anxiety is a common factor, and it's important to not ignore it. I still have residual moments, everybody does, but the trick, or rather the goal, is to work out how to manage and avoid these sometimes unexpected moments of anxiety.

Excited spikes, and nervous, panicked spikes are an overload on the nervous system, and for me, this has consequences every time. I see these as red flags, causing too much activity and triggering a cortisol reaction in my body. The overload is too much for me; the highs are too high, causing the lows to become unbearable, so I try to keep my nervous system happy and peaceful, with only calmness and positivity. Eliminating the spikes has therefore become my personal priority because then I am less likely to have a meltdown, burst into tears or, worse, want to lock myself away and hide until they pass.

Situations that cause me to spike include things like travel, being late and being unprepared or disorganised, but it can also be directly linked to my diet. For example, coffee can set me on edge, and certainly, as I entered peri-menopause, my tolerance for it lessened. But that is nothing like my alcohol intolerance; drinking even a little more than, say, a few glasses leaves me unable to sleep and panicked. Sugar is another culprit – too much and I feel unbalanced. In order to get to the bottom of all this I started a food journal, which enabled me to eliminate things that make me feel bad. This was the only way to track what was happening to my body as it changed. Keeping a food diary can be as simple as just jotting down in a small notebook everything you eat throughout the day. Having it close by, in the same way that you would carry a wallet, means you can keep a record and update it regularly, as needed. Of course, there are many apps for this, too, so if you do forget the diary, you can create a record on your phone or other device.

Speaking of which, one thing I would say about tech-nology, particularly social media, is that it is so easy to get overwhelmed by it. I sometimes find a simple email can cause my anxiety to spike, particularly if I am not prepared or in a good place to receive whatever news – good or bad – it is delivering. I also need to be careful not to overload my brain with too much information at one time. A good example is jumping from email to text to WhatsApp in close succession, checking Twitter, then moving to Instagram, then WhatsApp; before I know it, I have been skipping and scrolling for hours. This is not healthy for me, and I can't imagine it's healthy for anyone! I have had to force myself to take regular breaks from my phone, taking time to process each communication platform slowly and in a more considered way.

We can't always avoid information spikes in day-to-day life – particularly when we are working – but by keeping a handle on any adverse reactions, we can control the dramas, and make sure the unexpected turns are more easily processed. In the same way, I have set up a small list of things – 'user rules', if you like – such as not to have the phone in my hand for more than five minutes in any one hour to ensure my day goes smoothly.

WEIGHT GAIN

One of the most challenging aspects of getting older and reaching menopause has been sudden weight gain. It is sometimes quite shocking to notice the changes happening – the waistline spreading and the frustration of not being able to fit into some favourite jeans (or any of my wardrobe, in my case, when I was my heaviest) is not easy on the ego.

It's a known fact that our metabolisms slow down as we get older, and when you add hormones into the mix, causing all sorts of havoc, it's clearly a disaster waiting to happen.

For me, the weight gain felt like it came out of nowhere. In my head, I didn't think I had changed what I was eating (that's perhaps the first little white lie I have told you, because maybe I was drinking and eating more than I had previously). Feeling bigger affected my confidence massively and made me feel out of sorts and disconnected from myself. In all honesty, I felt a little disappointed with myself, too.

A moment which is ingrained in my memory was in April 2017, when George and I were back in Japan – our favourite country. We were in this stunning open-air *onsen* (Japanese hot spring), which was the perfect place for a picture that I could post on my grid. I was going to look like a water nymph at ease, bathing in the surrounding misty natural springs, and it would potentially get a lot of likes (something I think we all got a little too caught up in back then – maybe still to this day for me). George obliged, I sucked my belly in, arched my back and threw my arms in the air, convinced we were making art. But then, when I looked through the photos he had taken, I did not recognise the person I saw there. I honestly looked like someone completely different – less water nymph, more England Rugby Union player.

Now, I will be frank with you, George may be the worst Instagram husband ever, because the photos are never that good, but even I couldn't blame him for what I saw, as I scrolled through the selection. And that was the first moment of realisation – but I didn't do anything about it. I just sulked for a minute, then continued to eat all the deliciousness offered to me, starting with Japanese breakfasts (my favourite), consisting typically of a piece of salmon, sticky white rice, miso soup, pickles, tofu – basically, scrummy food, and a lot of it! I would continue throughout the day, consuming large lattes, sushi, more sticky white rice, soy sauce and lots of beer. Then I'd throw in some sweet treats, as I became obsessed with green tea KitKats. (Ahhh, man, they were good – but at 11 at night?!) I was basically eating my way around Japan.

I was clearly overindulging and enjoying my food just a little too much, but also eating the wrong types of food, bombarding my system with too much protein and way too much sugar and refined carbohydrates. And the thing is, for me this was not out of the norm; my body was usually able to deal with whatever I threw at it. But not this time.

I have always had a healthy relationship with food; I like it, it likes me, and we had lived harmoniously together for forty-five years – or at least until that moment. For those who have struggled with food throughout their lives and have had to work hard to control their intake and calorie limit, I worry that this phase could open old wounds and bring back a desire to be too restrictive. It is a very delicate balance; we need food for fuel, but too much is just not good, and if we don't put in the work to keep off the weight, it has the potential to stick.

I thought nothing more of the weight gain while I was travelling around Japan – after all, that's what happens on holiday – but it all came to a head one day that summer. I was with my best friend, who happens to be a gorgeous, blonde, six-foot supermodel, and I got the biggest wake-up call. I don't own scales and never have, as not only are they often misleading, I also know I have the tendency to be rather Bridget Jones and become obsessive, weighing myself all through the day, after each meal or pint of water, just to see. So I have always gone according to how my clothes feel. And that particular day I noticed that none of my clothes would fit. They were no longer just a bit snug – I couldn't get them over my hips. I was devastated and knew that I'd have to work even harder if I was to remain a stable, healthy weight.

I will be the first to admit that ageing and accepting that I am getting older haven't always sat well with me. I could feed you some bullshit about the fact that because I worked as a model for many years of my life I have always been judged on how I look, and to a certain degree that is, of course, true. But let's be honest – we are all guilty of being a little vain, and of scrutinising ourselves, finding fault with each part of us. We all torture ourselves with constant comparison, not helped by the unhealthy way we consume social media and magazine images, which are unrealistic and unachievable. The idea of perfection and not being enough infiltrates our subconscious day and night and is so damaging. There are triggers everywhere, too: the hideous overhead lighting that torments us in changing rooms, casting shadows and showcasing lumps and bumps that we'd swear weren't there before, causing us to balk at our reflections and run from there distraught. The shock when we open our phones and catch ourselves at the most unattractive angle. Or when we notice how even the skin on our knees isn't where it used to be. The way our metabolisms unfairly slow down and the weight piles on, as well skin and hair thinning and all that fun stuff. All these and more are part and parcel of this new phase of our lives.

Obviously, all this is harder to deal with on some days than others, but it all paled in comparison to what I was dealing with mentally in my early forties. It spiralled somewhat out of control for a few years, putting a strain on my relationship with George, and making work, and sometimes even leaving the house, a terrifying prospect.

In the end, I put on three stone through my perimenopausal years. Some people can put on more and others less, but that, for me, was too much. Getting rid of the extra stones was not easy and that's about the truth. I have had to work harder than ever, work out for longer and try many different types of activities in order to see a change. I have run, lifted weights and walked and walked for miles.

I've sweated and cried quite a lot, but I was determined to keep going. I still haven't lost all that weight, and I don't think I ever will. I lost two of the three stones, and I am coming to terms with the fact that it is what it is and now I can only try to tone everything up. I am a size or two bigger than I'd like, but I try not to let it concern me too much.

There is so much going on in this process, so you have to accept what you can and can't control and finding that balance is key. After all, life *is* about balance, and I happen to be one of those people who enjoys life to the full. Food brings me so much pleasure; I love eating, I love tasting new things. Food makes me so happy, cooking brings me so much joy, finding new restaurants and pubs – all of this, for me, is living, and that's what gives me a thrill. Date nights with George with a delicious bottle of wine gives me life and makes me very happy. And so I just remember that I have to keep it all in balance. If I have a large meal one day, I try to be careful the next. I try to limit what I am drinking to two glasses, and always try to make sure I exercise. Moderation in everything.

There are days when I am stricter with myself, and there are days when I say yes to that dessert. One size does not fit all when it comes to managing weight, but I do believe in intermittent fasting, fasting a few days a week or just having days when I practise strong self-control to check in with myself and realise what I need, what I want to achieve and what works for me. One thing I like to do a few times a week to give my system a break is to have dinner early, say around 6pm. I try to eat something light and nutritious – not too many processed carbohydrates, just lean protein and vegetables, pulses, or lentils – then I head off to bed without any alcohol and fast for around twelve to fifteen hours.

There is lots of research coming out proving that intermittent fasting helps to slow down the ageing process, and that it is positive for overall health, as well as managing the pile-on of pounds. Again, this approach isn't for everyone, and when we enter perimenopause and menopause it's a time to nourish our bodies, not deny them, so managing your weight is very individual and you need to find what works for you. As mentioned earlier, keeping a food diary, and noting not just what you eat but when you eat, is important because it also helps with monitoring how food or alcohol can impact sleep.

SOME WORDS FROM TIM SPECTOR ON THE SCIENCE BEHIND INTERMITTENT FASTING

The science on time-restricted eating as a practical way of introducing intermittent fasting is going from strength to strength. Our own ZOE research (the world's largest nutrition-science study) shows that simply giving your body and gut bugs a rest overnight can help improve energy and digestive symptoms and reduce cravings. Simply tuning into our natural sleep–wake cycle and eating in roughly the same window of time every day can have a really positive impact. I like to have my first meal around midday and dinner at 8pm, which works for me. Listen to your hunger cues and don't eat unless you're hungry: having breakfast when we wake up is no longer what the doctor orders.

So it's important to listen to your body as you eat, and observe its reactions to food. If you know that eating bread bloats you or doesn't sit well with your body, limit it. If you know sugary cocktails make you retain water and leave your skin dull and in breakouts, listen to your body – it is your greatest teacher and is capable of sending you the biggest signs. There will be foods that no longer agree with you, and drinks that aggravate your system. That's part of menopause and your hormones.

It has been documented that sugars and wine may also create a histamine reaction. The body sees these foods as an enemy trying to invade, and so it triggers a defence reaction that causes you to feel unwell, and you may, like me, have a funny turn as a result. Quite recently, I passed out in a restaurant (and I promise I wasn't drunk). Luckily, I was with George and some close friends, but it was still terrifying. I'd eaten a seafood dish, and it was like I had been spiked. What looked like an innocent mussel turned my stomach upside down. I know I am not allergic to them, although my stomach was off for a few days, but it reminded me that certain foods can start to be an issue or cause bloating, hives or a rash. It's simply because your body doesn't digest as well as it used to. It is, I am afraid, all trial and error, which is another reason why I'd advise starting a food diary.

The key thing to remember is that as we age, we just can't continue to bombard our systems and overload them in the same way, especially as we enter perimenopause.

Of course, the other mantra is hydration, hydration, hydration. Water is crucial for everybody, and it's something that most of us don't consume enough of. It is vital for all bodily processes: from supporting our circulatory systems to lubricating joints and eyes, flushing out toxins and helping our digestive systems. Not drinking enough water can cause headaches, lethargy, dizziness and lack of concentration, which are all things we experience in the menopause, too, so it's important to make sure you're always drinking enough water, about 6 to 8 glasses, throughout the day.

Drinking water can also make you feel fuller for longer, so sometimes when I feel hungry, I just grab a big glass of water. I usually have my reusable bottle with me – for those of you who know me from my Instagram lives, you'll recognise my trusty khaki-green one that's always by my side wherever I am in the world.

GUT: THE HORMONE CONNECTION

BY DR MEGAN ROSSI, DIETICIAN AND GUT-HEALTH SPECIALIST

It is obvious that gut symptoms are linked to our gut health, but what people are often surprised to learn is how much else is linked to our gut: from our metabolisms, to skin health and mental wellbeing.

You can also add hormones to that list, for yet another role of our all-powerful guts is to make and regulate hormones, including oestrogen. Without getting deep into the science, it's worth knowing that we all contain trillions of microbes – mostly bacteria, but also fungi, viruses and parasites – that synergistically live and work together to look after us. That is, if we look after them. This incredibly powerful community is known scientifically as our gut microbiota, and it's this that is able to influence circulating oestrogen levels, thanks to an enzyme that certain microbes produce called β-glucuronidase, which can turn inactive oestrogen into active oestrogen, recycling it from the gut back into the circulation. So it figures that looking after your gut health could help to ease a wide range of problems related to women's reproductive cycles, from polycystic ovaries to menopausal symptoms. And now we've finally got the science that backs up what I've been seeing in clinic for years: that better gut health tends to reduce hormonal distress.

Indeed, an imbalance in our gut microbiota, often referred to as dysbiosis, and a reduction in microbe diversity, has been shown to impact circulating oestrogen levels (both high and low, depending on which microbes dominate). This is thought to play a role in a range of common hormonal conditions, from polycystic ovarian syndrome (PCOS), endometriosis and infertility to menopause and breast cancer. Conversely, an abundant and diverse microbiota is more likely to keep oestrogen levels balanced, with the potential to reduce menopausal symptoms and conditions caused by imbalances in oestrogen levels. This may very well explain why in a one-year intervention study in over 17,000 menopausal women, those eating more fibre, including vegetables, fruit and soy, experienced a 19 per cent reduction in hot flushes compared to the control group. And one systematic review (where they pool together the individual trials on a topic – thirteen, in this case) found supplementing with specific probiotics could reduce symptoms of PCOS by reducing levels of hormones circulating in the blood and improving insulin resistance.

What's more, research from the UK Women's Cohort Study, which included over 900 women, showed that including more gut-loving foods, such as beans and pulses (high in prebiotics – fertiliser for our gut bacteria) and oily fish (high in anti-inflammatory omega-3) in your diet could delay the natural menopause by over four years.

KEEP MOVING

We cannot discuss food and weight gain without talking about movement.

I can't stress enough the importance of movement and how crucial this is for our bodies. So many of us lead sedentary lives due to office jobs, and with the lure of Netflix, bingeing box sets is a common after-work wind-down activity. However, sitting for long periods of time can not only exacerbate weight gain, but also create a whole host of potential postural problems. A sedentary life is so detrimental to our health because the body tightens and seizes up, causing the metabolism to slow down. It's one of the fastest ways to age us.

We are, quite simply, designed to move, and move we must – every day. Whether it's dancing in the kitchen while waiting for the kettle to boil (kitchen discos are a personal favourite of mine), going to a Pilates or a yoga class or getting off the bus or train one stop before your destination and walking the extra distance, there are many ways to get those 10,000 steps a day.

I know that there will be some days when the lack of motivation is real, or the overwhelming sense of exhaustion that comes with menopause just makes everything feel like a challenge. But I promise you, push through this, grab a big glass of water, eat some good food and get that booty moving, and your body, mind and soul will thank you for it.

WORK OUT REGULARLY

To keep the weight gain at bay, we need to increase our movement. It's that simple. We have to build muscle and bone density, which may protect against osteoporosis (according to Dr Louise Newson, we lose about 10 per cent of our bone mass in the first five years of the menopause). By exercising, we can ease any potential hip, knee or back issues as we get older, and it should also help to improve metabolism, which will help to maintain a healthy weight and cholesterol levels and reduce the risk of high blood pressure and heart disease. And let's not forget the mood-boosting release of endorphins that occurs during exercise.

Recently, I have started working out at the gym with a personal trainer. Now, I know that's not possible for everybody, and I appreciate I am very fortunate to be able to do it, but I see it as an investment – after all, health is wealth, and I am prepared to pay extra if it helps to keep me in good condition. I see my sessions with a trainer as a treat to myself in the same way that I would treat myself to a new handbag – except I have to pick one or the other, and I choose Paul, my trainer. I think it's important to reframe this in our minds: seeing exercise as a treat instead of a punishment might help to motivate you – which is why joining various classes at the gym that looked like fun seemed like a good idea to me. I really like classes that incorporate weightlifting, squats, kettlebell swings, bounding – basically, anything that really challenges me and makes me feel as if I am learning a new skill. The added bonus, of course, is that I am also strengthening my body. With each breath, each lunge and power pump, I can feel myself getting stronger and growing healthier.

It is crucial for us women to incorporate resistance and strength training into our exercise routines, as these build muscle, burn fat and increase metabolism, as well as supporting bone health during the menopause. You don't have to lift super heavy weights. In fact, everything you do in the gym should be done according to the plan you agree with your trainer at and after your induction. Don't worry, you're not going to get big and bulky, I promise, especially if you ask a professional trainer in your gym to assess you and recommend the best workout programme for you.

If joining a gym is not possible, there are many videos, books and even apps that you can use to start a regimen from your bedroom, and some of them are free. So even if you just hold the plank position for a few minutes every day, that's better than nothing. You can do resistance training at home, too, working out with water bottles or books and doing squats and star jumps – anything that involves moving or using your own body weight.

The effects of exercise are, of course, physical, but it can also impact our minds. I am buzzing when I leave the gym or a class, not least because I've had that sense of connection and community with other people. My favourite is Pilates classes – both mat Pilates and working on the reformer are great, especially if you have back issues or your core needs strengthening. It is always challenging, and you do get a good all-over body workout. The reformer has springs that create tension and options to make it easier or harder. We also incorporate hand weights, which we hold while doing lunges and squats for a proper full-body workout. If you have never exercised before, Pilates is fantastic.

Now, you may prefer yoga, in which case, you should do that – either in a class or online from the comfort of your home. This exercise is amazing for your system because that hour that you spend on yourself – time spent focused on you and your breathing – is going to calm the system down. I love yoga, although I will say that I have always found it very challenging. There are certain classes that are just so tricky and not for everyone, but it is important to try as many as possible until you find the one that best suits you and that you have fun doing. We have to be positive and challenge ourselves, especially as we get older. I quite often pour with sweat, regardless of what movement I am taking part in, as I am truly focused and I put in 100 per cent effort.

Having said that, some days I have to drag myself to a class, but I never ever regret it once I've finished. I always feel a huge sense of achievement and satisfaction and am extremely proud of myself to have taken that time out of my busy schedule to really nurture and nourish my mind and my body, away from my phone, away from life, just super focused on that moment.

This is so important for us ladies going into the peri-menopause and menopause. It's about slowing down our minds, our thoughts and our bodies by taking in more oxygen with each breath and calming the nervous system. We women are always running on empty, we're always going at full speed – we multitask and always say we're good at it, but is it good for *us*?

MOVEMENT IS MEDICINE

BY PAUL WEBB, STRENGTH AND MENTAL PERFORMANCE COACH

I was absolutely thrilled when Lisa asked me to contribute to this book by writing a section on exercise. When I discovered that she had chosen to call this section 'Movement is medicine', I was beside myself with excitement as, for me, it's the perfect title.

You see, movement *is* medicine. However, like all medicine, you need to get the right prescription and the correct dosage, otherwise it could prove detrimental to your efforts and, ultimately, your health. Now, let's get one thing out in the open straight away: we are designed to move and, as such, when we don't, we tend to suffer. The longer that non-movement continues, the more the suffering increases. Inactivity costs $117 billion in the United States alone, according to the Centers for Disease Control and Prevention, and the same body states that, 'Not getting enough physical activity can lead to heart disease – even for people who have no other risk factors. It can also increase the likelihood of developing other heart disease risk factors, including obesity, high blood pressure, high blood cholesterol, and type 2 diabetes.'

Also in the US, the Heart Foundation, in a 2011 study that documented 800,000 people and their sitting habits, found that people who sit the most, compared to people who sit the least, have a greater risk of disease and death, specifically:

- 112 per cent increased risk of diabetes
- 147 per cent increased risk of cardiovascular events, such as heart attack and stroke
- 90 per cent increased risk of death from cardiovascular events
- 49 per cent increased risk of death from any cause

These results alone should leave you with no confusion whatsoever over the fact that a lack of physical activity is probably the greatest threat to living a healthy, and maybe longer, life.

Just in case you're not completely sold yet, researchers from the K.G. Jebsen Centre for Exercise in Medicine at the Norwegian University of Science and Technology in Trondheim discovered that as little as three minutes of vigorous activity every day is linked to a 40 per cent lower risk of premature death in adults!

One of the reasons I've brought you all this research is because if a pharmaceutical company released a drug, with no side effects at all, and it decreased your overall risk of death from any cause significantly; if it also decreased your risk of type 2 diabetes, as well as dying from any cardiovascular event; if it helped reduce obesity, lowered blood pressure, lowered cholesterol, strengthened your bones, stopped the onset of sarcopenia (muscle and strength loss), significantly improved your mental health and improved not only your hormone profile, but helped immeasurably with the symptoms of perimenopause and menopause, would you take it? Of course, you would, right? Who wouldn't?

Well, such a 'drug' exists, except that it hasn't been rushed to market by a pharmaceutical company, but is yours for the taking, and that 'drug' is ... strength training! Strength training, or to give it its proper title, progressive resistance training, will do all the above. I don't say this because I've been a strength coach for thirty years (although that does give some weight to it); I say it because it's been backed by research for over twenty years now.

Does that mean that everyone should just lift weights, and everything will be just fine and dandy? Well, remember what I said at the beginning of this section? You have to get the prescription and dosage correct. Exercise prescription is never one-size-fits-all, more one-size-fits-one. Yes, we all benefit from strength training, but it is very much relative. How I strength-train as a 54-year-old man is different to how I train Lisa, and undoubtedly would be different to how I'd train you – but the philosophy behind the training is/would be the same.

I currently work out of Zone Six, a performance gym in Loughton, Essex, and have many perimenopausal and meno-pausal women as clients, as more and more women, thanks in part to people like Lisa shining a light on the subject, are taking back their power as they go through this natural change. But I think we should pause here one second to consider this vital piece of the menopausal puzzle ... What is happening to you is a natural and normal part of living as a woman. It isn't to be feared, judged or stressed over. The days when women had to 'suffer in silence' no longer exist, so you can feel empowered to take control of a very natural event and work with it, rather than battle against it!

In my experience as a coach who works with clients physically, mentally, emotionally and spiritually, I can categorically tell you that people suffer when they lack the information or knowledge to solve their problems. This section – and this book as a whole – is here, in your hands right now, full of the information and knowledge that you need to just apply. You are not alone, help is readily available, and you can feel empowered and confident over your body, your mind and your health.

So, with that said, let's dig into exercising through menopause, shall we? The very first thing I need to point out is that what may have worked for you in your twenties, your thirties, even in your early forties, will probably not work for you now. A common theme I see, and something that I know happened to Lisa, is that when the weight starts to go on, as it does in menopause, many people immediately either diet hard or start running. Others will hit the gym and choose to perform some sort of HIIT (high-intensity interval training) session.

There are other areas in the book that deal specifically with nutrition and hormones, so I won't address that here too much, but let's chat briefly about those exercise choices and why they fail during menopause. In a recent Finnish study (2021), researchers found that, compared to women in early perimenopause, those in late perimenopause had 10 per cent less muscle mass in their arms and legs. Also, the same study showed that late perimenopausal and postmenopausal women were more likely to have sarcopenia (involuntary muscle loss) than premenopausal or early perimenopausal women.

This is a common theme in similar research and shows that when women start to go through the menopause, they very quickly begin to lose muscle size, bone density, strength and power. This, added to the shift in hormone profile, very quickly lowers metabolism, and together, they will increase visceral fat, especially round the belly area – seemingly overnight!

What I'm often at pains to point out to clients is that muscle equals life, literally. A person's muscle mass, as I referenced previously, is inversely associated with an earlier risk of death. Adults with low muscle mass are more likely to die early than those with more muscle, so this makes menopause a key time of life to improve your odds of both vitality and longevity by adding as much muscle mass to your frame as possible.

The problem that hampers this process in so many people is that they choose an exercise modality that does little to improve their muscle mass; for example, they run, or they do a HIIT class. Now, in and of themselves, these are perfectly fine. I often recommend that people use many different forms of exercise for a well-rounded approach to their fitness and health, so will often add some running and a HIIT session to a progressive strength programme. However, as I keep saying, it really depends on the individual and, if you are going through menopause, running and a HIIT class will increase your levels of cortisol dramatically, which will have the double whammy of reducing your muscle mass (and therefore your metabolism) and actually increasing your belly fat!

The reason for this is that there is an abundance of cortisol receptors in the stomach area, so if you perform an exercise that creates a lot of stress on the body, as do steady-state cardio (like running) and very high-intensity training (like HIIT), you may lose a little weight initially, but you will very quickly plateau and then start to actually put weight on.

This is exactly what happened to Lisa, and it's a story I've heard from so many women who have tried to shift weight in this way.

If you only take one lesson from this section, then please let it be this: you cannot fight against your body and win. You will lose every single time. So, if you want to enjoy the best vitality, health, wellness and strength as you go through menopause, you are going to need a multi-faceted process – one which includes good-quality sleep, optimal hydration and eating nutrient-dense foods (staying away from anything processed, and that means processed plant-based foods as well).

That is your foundation. From there, you want to make sure you are active every day – so go for a walk, do some gardening, take the dog out, go for swim or a yoga class, and then take good advice and begin a progressive strength-training programme designed to get you stronger, build a little muscle, keep your bones strong, help your hormones and, really importantly, help your mental health!

I cannot ethically write your personal strength programme for you here, as I know nothing about you or your training and medical history; however, some advice to consider is that you want to make sure your training programme covers the fundamental movement patterns we all move with. That means you want to bend or hinge from the hips, squat, lunge, push, pull and rotate (or perform an anti-rotation movement like a side plank) in each training session, or across a training week.

It sounds a big undertaking, but in actuality, it's quite simple. This doesn't mean, of course, that you'll find it easy, but with a little bit of advice, and some practice and consistency, you will find that the results will come, and that going through menopause needn't be feared as it may be for you right now.

CHANGE YOUR MINDSET AND WORK ON ACCEPTANCE

Acceptance is something we must all strive for. When we get to the point where we can accept who we are, life becomes a lot easier. It doesn't mean we just give up – far from it; I see acceptance and practising it as an act of evolving, of growing and maturing, of acknowledging the challenges that have been, the ebb and flow of life and what it has thrown at us. We are learning to love our battle scars, if you will.

I have started to view acceptance as a state of mind not dissimilar to that of a Buddhist monk. It's a zen-like quality, whereby you try to find yourself as you start to get older. You learn to glide through life, to not sweat the small stuff, almost like learning to meditate. I am not saying it's easy, and for any of you who do meditate, you'll know that it takes practice, years, even, to perfect. Sometimes, on those low-mood days, when nothing is going well, your brain can short-circuit and revert back to you picking holes in yourself and finding things to punish yourself with – whether with the unkind, hurtful, nasty words you mutter under your breath when you look in the mirror, or through the self-harm you indulge in by eating and drinking too much, or by savagely picking pimples and biting fingernails to the quick or by scrolling through

Instagram and comparing yourself and your life to other people's. On those days, and on most days, in fact, I try to view myself through rose-tinted glasses, a soft-focus lens that blurs the edges of my reality. The fact that my eyesight is also going makes it so much easier – I'm sure it is nature's way of being kind! It's only when I get a glimpse in the magnifying mirror when I do my eye make-up that I get the cold, harsh reality of how I really look – but even then, I take that with a pinch of salt as no one ever sees me THAT close, thankfully.

When I say practise acceptance, I don't mean you should ignore the extra weight or the new lumps and bumps that you have started to accumulate, or the changes in your hair and skin. It would be remiss not to acknowledge the passing of time, the fine lines of wisdom and the pigment in your hair disappearing. And I am embracing all these wholeheartedly. Although perhaps that is not entirely true, as if it were, I wouldn't be cover- ing God's organic highlights (the grey) with tint or be slathering myself in lotions and potions having upped my 'at-home' beauty regime.

The truth is, I enjoy looking good and these little beauty treatments help me to feel really good, plus I do enjoy taking care of myself and have always been a self-con- fessed beauty junkie. Looking and feeling good, for me, equal confidence – and that is something I am passionate about for all of us.

So, I am not saying just give up and accept getting older. What I mean is, you must dig a little deeper and start to have an abundance of self-love and self-acceptance for everything you've been through, for how utterly incredible your body is, for everything it's done for you throughout the years. You need to allow yourself to be proud of your achievements, for getting through the hard times, the happy times, the sad times and the times when you haven't been kind to your body.

I try not to have any regrets – it is such a waste of energy – but when I think about it, I have really taken my body for granted over the years. Put it this way: my body has most definitely NOT been my temple! But that's life; I drank everything possible – not in an out-of-control alcoholic way, but I certainly tried every different type of alcohol, adding all sorts of hideously calorific, vile, sugary fizzy drinks. I smoked and partied my booty off, and I had a LOT of fun doing it. I also tried every fried option on every menu, ate all the takeaways and chocolate biscuits and salt and vinegar crisps were a breakfast staple of mine for many years. (I cannot believe I am admitting that!) And, weirdly, my body allowed me to do all of this. I even seemed to get away with it – no hangovers, no heartburn or weight gain. I would just burn it all off and bounce right back!

Oh, how things have changed. It is payback time now, and as my dad has always said to me: 'Lisa, it always catches up with you in the end, love'. How right he is. I am so thankful I had those times, as they certainly were carefree and fun, but I am now happy with my new-found love, appreciation and respect for my body and for all it has done and continues to do for me every day.

When I say I have a sense of self-acceptance, I think we all must realise that we don't look like our 25-year-old selves – and that's quite simply because we are no longer twenty-five. And thank God for that, because even though my skin was flawless and my arse was firm, that was a tricky time. It was a challenging period when I was trying to find my feet, discover who I was and determine what I wanted to do. I had zero concept of any sort of self-worth, and I used to pick holes in every single little area of my body and my life, comparing myself endlessly to others and allowing in toxic people.

I have now got to a place where I really like who I am. I can appreciate my good qualities and focus on them more. I also really … wait for it … love my body! I like how I look.

Of course, it's not the younger body I used to know – the firm, smooth, even-skinned, skinny Minnie that could wear anything (even though I didn't, and was so self-conscious). I certainly did not appreciate my body back then, or what I looked like, and I don't think any of us did. But looking back at old photos, oh, my goodness! I often think, this is as good as it's going to get, and in twenty years, I'll look back at the 50-year-old me and feel the same way. However, I will say that this version of me is strong and healthy. I have learned to love and accept that with the passing years, not only am I fighting gravity in all areas of my body and face, but it's also just a part of life; things start to sag, and we also expand every year ever so slightly (or not so slightly, depending on consumption and lifestyle). And, of course, stress plays a huge part in ageing, too.

I am also battling mentally with time. We all are. It is going far too quickly. So, the sooner we can start to connect with who we really are – with the innermost part of ourselves – the sooner we can just get on with it. I am hoping that with this midlife manual by your side, including all my tips and tricks, you can stop wasting time worrying about silly insignificant things and get out there, make the changes, put in the work, get the help, advice and back-up, communicate your feelings, vocalise your needs and be a support network to the people who need you. Then we can all start to live our best fucking lives.

FINDING BALANCE

It's not always a perfect day for me, I'll admit that, and constant work is required for me to ensure I am in a good headspace, and that I am taking the utmost care of my mind and my body.

One thing I'm learning as I get older is that the brain needs balance and a healthy, happy environment, which means doing things that make us happy, that keep us calm, sometimes pressing reset and avoiding those triggers – whether that's people, places or situations. Life will constantly throw us curveballs, and while we can't always dodge these, we can change the way we react to them and learn to respond more calmly and be more in control, taking back ownership of the situation.

I practise a lot of gratitude daily – for the life I live, for the love I have, the love that I receive and the people I have in my life – the close-knit friendships, the family members, all the love and the laughter I have with the people I adore spending time with. Small things and small wins cultivate gratitude for the bigger things. I give deep love and respect for who I am, what I have been through and that I live to tell this tale. And I have hopes, dreams and aspirations for the future, as you will, too. Just stick with me …

Starting the day with mindfulness, breathwork (see page 155) or meditation – even just for ten minutes – will help to ground you and get you into a good headspace first thing, so that when any crap comes your way, you will be like a superhero with a force field around you, protecting you. And practising these things daily will help you to be the happiest, most resilient woman with the most kick-ass attitude. I promise you that armed with that attitude, acceptance will follow.

A happy outlook, a positive mindset, that get up and go and joie de vivre are infectious, and you can spread the love just by being the best version of you. I know we all get thrown out of kilter by stuff that happens. And then, if you add the fluctuation of hormones, weight-gain, heartbreak, disappointment and exhaustion into the mix, you start to feel frazzled and beyond repair. So you need to make big changes, reframe your approach and realise that getting older is a privilege. A good attitude and a sense of humour go a hell of a long way.

Life can be hard. We don't get a manual on how to navigate it, and some days it's harder to pick ourselves up off the ground. But you are still you. Yes, you may be viewed differently by a society that has a weird and twisted attitude to ageing, but that shouldn't shape how you feel about yourself, and it doesn't mean you can't be the change and, in turn, make the change. Plus, I have learned that there is something so liberating about finally giving zero fucks to what people think of me; I wasted so many years caring a little too much about this.

EVERYBODY NEEDS GOOD FRIENDS

The thing about getting older is that sometimes it feels like we're running out of time, and as a result, we become very protective of that time, particularly with what we share with others. I have always been blessed with a solid group of friends, but sometimes it can be difficult when we snap at each other or treat each other in ways that don't feel right.

People can be mean, can treat us badly and say hurtful things. Words are so hard to forget, and the scars run very deep. Sometimes, too, when we hear hurtful things over and over, we start to believe them, and this is dangerous. If someone makes you uneasy, or if a friend is unnecessarily cruel or unkind or you start to pick up on even a hint of negativity, then look for signs that maybe they're going through something. It is possible that they are simply having a tough time. I always give the benefit of the doubt and look for solutions to help with their problem.

However, it's a sad fact of life that we do outgrow people, and that people change, and that is when we must take control and no longer give them the energy they feed on. If a friend or someone close to you can't see that they're directly hurting you and they are repeatedly negative and unkind to you, then as harsh as it sounds, you may need to cut them out. You will always, *always* get a gut instinct or an inkling about a person or a situation, and at this stage of your life, it's important to act upon that. This is a time to protect yourself from triggers that could unravel your peace of mind, adding to your already fragile state and leaving you feeling unsupported and lacking in confidence. You will immediately feel a sense of relief when you no longer have any communication with the person in question and don't need to spend precious nights out with them, experiencing their draining effect. See ya!

To even get to the point where you are strong enough to do this and where you are attracting the right kind of people, you must start liking or, rather, loving who you are, appreciating that you can bring a lot to the table, being proud of what you have achieved and of who you are. That way, you will only let good people, worthy people, into your life. There is simply no room for time wasters, naysayers or narcissistic people. Good vibes only!

Think of it in the same way that you would if you had an injury or an illness, or if you were undergoing any medical treatment. Rehabilitation requires a lot of strength, involving both physical and emotional effort and determination and, more importantly, unwavering support from people you love. So, you need to surround yourself with good, solid relationships and people who are there to support you and want you to do well and succeed – people who will fight your corner. It may only be one or two solid friends you can rely on, and that's OK. My circle of friends has shrunk over the years. Getting into my late forties and early fifties, I worked out who was there for me, who had my back, who I could call in the middle of the night when the shit hit the fan and who would take my call at 2am and talk to me. A true friend is someone who offers no judgement whatsoever, someone who's there to wrap their arms around you, to listen and give good advice, regardless of the mistakes you've made or the stupid things you've said.

BE YOUR OWN CHAMPION

Knowing that you have a close-knit group of individuals who love and accept you – adore you, even – is truly empowering. However, this will mean nothing if you find it hard to love and accept yourself. You would never speak horribly to your friends, or say hurtful or unkind words, so why do it to yourself?

I have said some vile, hurtful and nasty things to myself. I remember the day so clearly when I realised I had put on three stone, and I sat on the floor just sobbing my heart out. I was trying on clothes because I was due to go out, and when nothing fitted me and a big pile of clothes started gathering around me, I just broke down.

I have been unkind to myself physically as well. At times, I have neglected to look after me, and that's something I am determined to really hammer home to others. This is the time for you to be your own best friend. Be your own champion and give yourself the same support, love and respect that you bestow on others. It's OK to be critical, because that keeps you moving forwards and can lead to growth and development, but within that, be fair and kind to yourself.

For me, it all goes back to the importance of maintaining balance at this time of life. When the apple cart topples over and I take on too much or am burning the candle at both ends, consumed by stress and worry, suffering from not enough sleep and not practising my meditations, it can all go to absolute shit – and that's when I have a monumental meltdown (or a stage-five meltdown, as I have started to call it). This is where the red mist descends, I can't see straight, and I almost have an out-of-body experience of anger that's more out of control and aggressive than anything I've known before.

Listen, for years we girls have been known for our brilliant multitasking abilities. We say yes to everything and everyone and demonstrate our superior skills by juggling it all, being in a million different places at once, pushing ourselves to the absolute limit and basically being superhuman and proud of it. Sadly, as we get older, our fuses start to shorten, and we start to experience burnout. And speaking for myself, I have a much lower tolerance threshold for people and experience huge amounts of frustration if even the tiniest thing goes wrong; this will trigger me, lighting the end of that stick of dynamite, detonating an almighty explosion.

So, this is a time for us to recognise what is happening, and to try to nip it in the bud before the explosion happens – to make those adjustments that take us back to a state of calm, to get back in control and achieve a sense of balance.

For so many years, I was running on empty and I just can't do that any more – or if I do, there are major consequences. My whole world almost collapses, and I feel so out of control. On these days, and when my sleep has been impacted and I haven't been moving my body or taken time out for me, my equilibrium gets totally skewed and then it all starts to go very wrong. I eat too much of the wrong foods (mostly sugar) to compensate for the lack of sleep and I cave in to cravings and drinking to excess, my mind quickly becoming scrambled. In these moments, I don't recognise myself, and I go into a very dark, horrible place. And that's when I need to press the reset button. Quickly.

However, often that's easier said than done. Because when I am in the throes of a stage-five meltdown no one can talk me down off the ledge, not even my long-standing and most patient, loving and caring best friend and partner for life, George. I go into self-destruct mode, utterly distraught at life and myself. I honestly turn into a total psychopath. All my healthy hacks fly away, and I desperately try to rein it all back in.

The only way I have managed to keep ahead of the curve to stay steady is by practising my daily breathwork. This calms my nervous system and eliminates any worry and anxiety I may have going into the day. I make sure I get some exercise in – whether it's a good, brisk walk around the block, up to the supermarket or into the forest or a

Pilates or resistance-training class. I try to push myself and therefore prevent any negativity descending.

I find that writing lists is the best way to keep on top of what I need to do, as well as going more slowly and not saying yes to everything and everyone just to appease them. For example, if I'm not able to meet someone, or feel it may trigger me into a mild panic as I have already enough to do, I don't do it. It's honestly not worth it. There is immense power in saying no, not stretching yourself beyond your limits. Boundaries give you a fantastic sense of authority; by drawing these lines you can have more control over and insight into those warning signs of doing too much and pushing too hard.

For instance, I know that when I drink too much too regularly, without any breaks, it's not going to agree with me. I had an eight-month pause from booze back in 2021, which I found surprisingly easy, and the benefits were truly incredible: I slept for longer periods and more deeply, experiencing much more restorative sleep. I woke up feeling refreshed and energised, and I lost weight, too, which made me very happy. Many people don't realise the calorific content of a glass of wine or a pint of beer – it is literally liquid cake. I also find that when I don't drink, I also eat much less in general, I think more clearly and I have more energy. In fact, as I write this, I am thinking, Why the hell don't I just stop again? I would thoroughly recommend it to anyone whose trigger is booze – whether that extra glass of wine turns you into a crazy person, those yummy margaritas give you anxiety and cause you to wake up in the middle of the night or if you are struggling with your weight. Be honest with yourself. If alcohol is impacting your life and causing the balance to topple, please either give it a wide berth for a while or just quit completely.

SLEEP

Sleep is vital for recovery and being able to function well the next day. And during menopause, it can be severely impacted, in turn impacting energy levels, as well as diet and exercise.

I've now got my sleep back on track, but it took a little while and I had to adopt some new wind-down techniques, but now I sleep so well. I have a routine of going to bed and waking up at the same time each day, and I practise a few sleep rituals. Here are some of my sleep hacks to help you get into healthy habits and really embrace the idea of good sleep hygiene. Try them and see what works for you:

MAGNESIUM – this mineral is great to take at bedtime to help relax body and mind, and it has the added benefit of helping to heal the body after exercise and aiding in muscle recovery.

5-HYDROXYTRYPTOPHAN (5-HTP) – a mood regulator that helps raise serotonin levels in the brain, this has a positive effect on sleep and anxiety. I find it helps me to switch off, so it is great to take at night before bed. Both George and I take this.

MELATONIN – I take this from time to time as it helps me to fall asleep more quickly and stay asleep. I was introduced to it when I was travelling, as it is amazing for jetlag, although it's sometimes hard to get in the UK without a prescription. It's basically a hormone that occurs naturally in the body that helps to regulate our circadian rhythms. It isn't something to take long term, but it can be beneficial from time to time when you are travelling or when your sleep is particularly out of whack. I find it helps, but please make sure, as with everything, to discuss with your doctor before taking it.

CBD – I have started to use CBD sprays, as well as drops. The drops work for me, but they may not be everyone's cup of tea. I use these at night-time and also have them in my handbag for any situations that may occur during the day, like being stuck in traffic or delayed on a train or anything that causes added stress. I use it to reinstate zen and calm into the moment, along with my trusty bottle of Rescue Remedy. There are some CBD products that include calming herbs as well, which I like to use at night.

AROMATHERAPY PILLOW SPRAYS, BODY SPRAYS, OILS AND LOTIONS – whether you roll it on your temples or wrists or spray it all over you, scent can anchor you in a night-time routine and help to quieten the mind, so that you can centre yourself and get into a good space before bed.

SLEEPY-TIME TEAS – these are good to drink an hour or so before bedtime, as they usually contain calming herbs such as valerian, chamomile and lavender, while some contain more calming nourishing herbs like ashwagandha and shatavari, which are great for us ladies, either at night or throughout the day. (See more on these in the alternatives to HRT section, page 135.)

TURN OFF SCREENS – stay off all screens for at least an hour before bed. That includes the TV, sadly. The blue light that is emitted from the devices is overstimulating for your brain, so make sure you set an alarm to include some downtime, either listening to music or reading, before you head off to bed.

SET THE SCENE – a dark, cool room is best for sleeping in, and make sure the lighting is low to kickstart levels of melatonin (see page 130). Make sure your bed is comfortable; a decent mattress is imperative, and while this is an investment, as a good one can be expensive, we do spend a lot of time in our beds, so it must be an enjoyable and comfortable place to be. Breathable sheets are more important than ever with the perimenopause and menopause years, and this can be a game changer in keeping your temperature regulated throughout the night, especially if those night sweats and flushes come thick and fast.

EYE MASKS AND EAR PLUGS – these are brilliant for the light sleeper, like me, as they block out sound and early-morning light and encourage a deeper, longer restful period. For anyone suffering with tinnitus, there is an app that plays white noise to help quieten the ringing with whooshing or wave sounds. There is also an alarm clock that can also play different sounds.

TECHNOLOGY – I also have become obsessed recently with a little bit of technology – my Oura ring. I have my best friend, Michele, to thank for this, as it was a generous birthday gift. It monitors not only your sleep, but your steps and heart rate when you are active, as well as your oxygen levels. The exciting part for me is it can work out and analyse how many hours of deep and REM sleep

I've had and how long I've been asleep for, as well as how long it took me to get to sleep. It is basically like my health app on steroids, as it does pretty much everything. It also has meditations that you can do – wake-up ones, winding-down, destressing, the lot. You pay a monthly charge to sync the app to the ring and off you go. The fitness app linked to the smartphone is fantastic as well. It is so good for keeping an eye on how many steps you are doing, as well as for using the meditations, workouts and mindfulness suggestions it offers.

I try not to beat myself up if I do have a late night or if my sleep has been affected or interrupted, instead consoling myself that my brain is an incredible thing and it will get me through the next day, then I can charge up the following night and get back on track.

Something else to consider is that you shouldn't compare your sleeping hours with anyone else's. We all need different amounts of sleep, but what is most important is to implement good sleep hygiene for yourself, and that means using the techniques and tips I have mentioned already, as well as making sure you have a good routine that you can stick to. It will soon become second nature. And don't forget to pack your sleep essentials whenever you travel or have a night away.

HRT

The data has shown that over the last six years, demand for HRT has risen, which, I believe, is in part due to incredible women like Mariella Frostrup, Meg Mathews and Davina McCall, who have documented their own stories with the menopause and perimenopause and got people talking out loud about an issue that has been whispered about for so long. This uptake of HRT surprised the pharmaceutical industry so much that there were shortages, which meant women who were on HRT or who had fought to have it prescribed were struggling to access it for a while.

Although HRT is discussed more openly today and considered as an option more often than previously, there is still much controversy around it, with many women too afraid to take it and doctors wary of prescribing it. This is due to some studies in the early 2000s that suggested that HRT gives you cancer. These stats were very misleading and proved to be wrong, but panic ensued because of these claims and many women were either too scared to continue taking HRT or were taken off it by their doctors, regardless of their medical situation or condition. What is really important to note is that this included women who had undergone oophrectomy (removal of their ovaries). This is called surgical menopause, and as the hormones are removed instantly the withdrawal of access to HRT left some of these women at risk of debilitating symptoms and other diseases.

HRT used to be taken in pill form. This would have been a combined pill containing oestrogen and progestogen. However, these days there are so many different preparations; oestrogen is mostly taken through the skin through gels and sprays, and there are pessaries, pills and creams that can be used, too.

HRT HERBAL ALTERNATIVES

If you are concerned about taking HRT, there are some alternative supplements available, some of which I dabbled with before being prescribed the correct HRT, and a few I still like to take. Some women swear by these, not only to alleviate menopausal symptoms, but to help with other wellness and health issues, too, while others (like me) prefer to use them alongside their HRT or instead of it.

There are mixed reviews from women as to whether any of these herbal remedies are effective, so I would say to try for yourself, remembering to incorporate the other aspects of wellness and that I have already discussed in this book – breathwork, movement, meditation, mindfulness. Used in combination, they can all help.

Please make sure to do your research to see if any of these herbal supplements may interfere with other types of medication you are taking and, of course, if you are pregnant, do take extra care.

Remember, nothing is a silver bullet, so whatever you choose should be part of a 360-degree approach. Consistency is key to getting back on track, thriving and owning your life again.

SAGE – I drank sage tea when my flushes were at their worst, and I found that it did help me a little. Sage is also available in oral supplement form, which evidence has shown to be slightly more effective. Try for hot flushes and night sweats.

ASHWAGANDHA – this is known as an adaptogen, which helps to balance hormonal symptoms and reduce stress and anxiety. It can also help to boost stamina and energy levels, as well as concentration.

MACA – a Peruvian root vegetable known as a superfood, maca is high in iron and iodine to help promote healthy cells and give us energy. It is also supposed to be good for hormone health, keeping metabolism on track and helping with libido and stress. Men can also take this, as it helps with erectile dysfunction and increases libido in both sexes.

SHATAVARI – this is a great herb for us ladies. It is oxidant-rich, which is great for skin and overall health, and it helps with all areas of female health, as it regulates hormones. I have read that it helps with metabolism as it contains saponins, which help the body burn fat more effectively.

CBD – this is not a menopause cure by any means, but I find CBD helpful to control some of the anxiety and stress I feel day to day as I have got older. It helps to calm the cortisol levels in my body when fight or flight response causes me to have a meltdown. I find it comforting to have it in my handbag or nearby to take the edge off the days when life gets on top of me. I also like to take CBD drops orally to help me wind down at night.

HRT – HORMONE REPLACEMENT THERAPY

BY DR NAOMI POTTER, BRITISH MENOPAUSE SOCIETY ACCREDITED SPECIALIST

This is the standard treatment for perimenopause and menopause symptoms. Essentially, it is replacing the hormones that were there before but are no longer. Replacing them normally helps remove symptoms and makes you feel better.

There are three hormones typically prescribed: oestrogen, progesterone and testosterone.

Oestrogen

Replacing oestrogen is the mainstay of treatment. It can be replaced via the skin (our preferred, safest route) in the form of patches, gels and sprays, or through oral tablets. Tablets can be good for ease of use. It can also be used in the form of topical cream, gel, ring or pessary for urinary or vaginal symptoms.

Progesterone

This is normally used for women with a womb to protect the lining from the additional oestrogen. It can be taken as a capsule, a patch, as part of a tablet combined with oestrogen, or as a Mirena coil. It is important to use progesterone as well as oestrogen, because taking oestrogen on its own for a prolonged time can increase the risk of cancer in the lining of the womb.

Testosterone

As a hormone that can decline in menopause, we sometimes replace this if it is low and using oestrogen doesn't improve symptoms, particularly that of a low libido.

HRT risks and benefits

HRT can help maintain bone density and cardiovascular health; there is also evidence that it can lower mortality rates and emerging evidence of its benefits to brain function. It also very much helps to alleviate sometimes debilitating symptoms.

Two decades ago, there was some new evidence that suggested HRT was strongly linked to breast cancer, clots, heart disease and stroke. As a result, many women stopped HRT or did not start it. Since then, these conclusions have been re-evaluated and we now understand it is much safer than we thought. Many women still fear HRT, but most recent evidence suggests that the newer HRT with body-identical progesterone is very safe, with a minimal increased risk of breast cancer. In fact, drinking two glasses of wine a night increases the risk of breast cancer more than taking HRT.

'Oestrogen dominance' and 'adrenal fatigue' are terms that are used in some spheres of alternative medicine. However, they are (as yet) unproven terms often used as diagnoses after expensive, unnecessary blood tests have been performed.

- **OESTROGEN DOMINANCE** – women can be told they are producing too much oestrogen and/or too much cortisol; if you are diagnosed with oestrogen dominance, please ask to see a British Menopause Society accredited specialist for accurate advice.
- **ADRENAL FATIGUE** – any woman with adrenal pathology should see an endocrinologist for an evidence-based diagnosis.

Part Three

We're Just Getting Started

This is my favourite part of the book, and it was the most fun to write. Why? Because this is where we start to take ownership of how we want to live our lives by considering everything we have been through so far. In my case, this was years of unprocessed hurt and disappointment and coming to terms with how my life now looks as opposed to how I once imagined it would. This reshaping and reframing of my future was essential in getting me to this stage and I really hope that the first two parts of the book have opened up a window for you to reflect on yours.

What I will aim to do in the next few pages is show you how wonderful life can be with a little bit of work. I will talk about some tried-and-tested ways to lift my mood, set me up for the day and nurture and love myself more. We're going to talk mindfulness, lots of self-care and gratitude. We're going to get into some sexy time – or lack of, in my case (anybody else with me? Just me? OK), as well as skin, nutrition and celebrating how fucking fabulous it is to be us and to acknowledge that we are exactly where we are meant to be right now.

SELF-CARE

Let's look at self-care. What does that mean to you? What do you do that constitutes self-care?

Let's be clear. Self-care isn't being selfish. It's an integral part of living well, of honouring ourselves, listening to our minds and bodies and knowing what we really need. I can hear you saying to yourself as you read this: 'I don't have time for self-care'. Well, you do, and it's so important that we all *make* time for it. As I have said you can't give from an empty cup, and often our cups are bone dry because we haven't replenished them for a while. And that means we can't give back to anyone in our lives.

The importance of self-care really became clear to me during the Covid pandemic. The idea that we were to stay at home and not go anywhere or do anything except walk for an hour a day was so strange. We needed to look after our minds, to protect and shield ourselves from the uncertainty and anxiety around us over what was happening in the world – the severity of a virus that had the potential to kill us or have long-lasting complications, the daily news conference punctuating each day – and cope with being restricted to staying within four walls the majority of the time. We were responsible for keeping ourselves healthy and for doing whatever we could to enable that.

The first few days – and maybe for some of you, weeks – it felt like a novelty staying at home, working from home, going about life in general more slowly. Some days, even getting dressed seemed unnecessary. Why not just lounge around? After about a week into lockdown, though, and with both George and I recovering from Covid, we realised the importance of getting up, taking a shower and getting dressed into something other than PJs. It aided our recovery and made us feel human again.

The rituals of each morning – bathing, hair washing, applying a little make-up (for me) and feeling ready for the day – all helped to create a sense of health and routine for us. The daily walks became our lifeline, as we began to truly appreciate where we lived, grateful for the forest surrounding us and our outside space. We tidied the house and had a thorough clear out of cupboards and drawers, which gave us a sense of clarity as we had too much clutter. I started to look through bags of products and half-used toiletries, and really took my time to delve and explore my 'at-home' self-care.

That is when I started my Self-care Sunday series on Instagram, which was not only an outlet for me but also how I connected with so many of you. It was an important time for us all, as we couldn't see anyone – not even our loved ones.

The series started with basic beauty, addressing all the things we would usually go to professionals for – such as colouring our hair (which I did not adopt, instead opting for home products that helped to temporarily cover my grey and shampoos to tone down the brassiness of my colour), and also finding products to remove gel nail polish safely. Essentially, it was about sharing lots of basic beauty hacks to see us through, as none of us knew how long we would be living in lockdown.

I started to explore and share more mental and physical wellness tips by speaking to experts on facial massage and crystal healing and doing live Pilates classes and workouts. There were some extremely positive moments throughout that time, and I for one managed to feel a sense of balance.

That was almost three years ago, and a lot has changed since then. But I would say my menopause symptoms were at their worst in 2020. Like so many of you, I also had to cope with life-changing symptoms, and it has been a challenge to say the least. I am not sure if it was the pandemic, coincidence or just the fact that, unbeknown to me, I'd moved through my perimenopause into full-blown menopause. Subconsciously, self-care became my anchor to get me through the day.

I am now most definitely postmenopausal, as it has been over two years since my last bleed. I need to work hard to put myself first and make sure I am taking all the necessary steps to keep myself well – mentally, physically, emotionally and spiritually. These are what I consider to be my four pillars of health.

It is so clear when I'm not taking care of myself, as everything gets tipped out of balance and I start to spiral out of control – and quickly. As I said earlier, if something goes even a little bit wrong, or something changes or is not how I was expecting it to go, I can totally overreact, become completely overwhelmed and tumble down a worry wormhole. If I don't address my daily self-care rituals at this point, it has a negative impact on everything in my life.

As soon as I stop taking care of my mind it impacts everything. I might then require an extra cup of coffee because I feel I am not focused, and that might sharpen me up. And then, of course, I drink too much and become jittery. As I mentioned before, stimulants in whatever shape may spike our cortisol levels – something us ladies entering this time of our lives need to be very mindful of.

Wellness is a 360-degree approach, encompassing all aspects of our lifestyle. The reason I recorded my podcast series 'Get Lifted' was to address these fundamental basics, my four pillars, vital components that should be in equilibrium and harmony. When one is off kilter, it will affect the others.

SPIRITUAL: Taking care of your soul. Are you trusting your intuition? Are you protecting yourself from other people's negative energies? Are you checking in with yourself on a deeper level?

MENTAL: Taking care of your mind. Are you repeating negative thought patterns? Are you deliberately trying to sabotage your own happiness? Are you being cruel to yourself?

PHYSICAL: Taking care of your body. Are you moving enough? Are you getting your steps in? Are you stretching, going outside in nature and taking in big lungfuls of fresh air?

EMOTIONAL: Taking care of yourself. This one embodies all three. You can't have one without the other; they are, in my opinion, all interconnected.

My mental wellbeing impacts my physical wellbeing, and when these are both good, together they stabilise my emotional wellbeing, which means I'm more in tune and aware of my spiritual wellbeing.

SPIRITUAL WELLBEING

You might be confused when I talk about spiritual wellbeing, and some of you may think it's a little woo-woo, but I think we must be conscious and aware that everything is energy. It surrounds us, and it's not always understood, but we are energy, and there are bad energies out there, too. You know what it's like when you walk into a room and there's just a weird feeling that you get? Well, that is your intuition telling you, warning you, alerting you to be aware; that is your spiritual protection, the energy you send off in response to the energy you are receiving.

I have always been attracted to the more esoteric, mystical side of life, believing that in the scheme of things we are so small, so insignificant. Astrology and the astrometry fascinate me, as do crystals, past-life conversations and the possibility of reincarnation.

I used to always carry a small piece of rose quartz in my bra, on the left-hand side, so it was close to my heart, because I found this gave me a sense of protection, and when I was in any doubt about a situation, worried about going to a particular place or starting a new job, this would bring me comfort. While writing this, I am holding three jellybean-shaped crystals called fluorite, which are meant to be cleansing and energising. They also calm a chaotic mind (hello!) and promote free thinking. Just what I need to finish this book.

George called me a white witch when we first got back together, because of my love of crystals, angel cards, smudging sage and palo santo around the house and burning incense and frankincense. Smudging freshens up the flow within your home, clearing stagnant energy and cleansing the space, especially if anyone has been into the house and created bad vibes or left you with an uncomfortable feeling. Pretty much each day we will burn either frankincense or incense – or both – and we always have candles burning, creating a sense of calm and a lovely atmosphere. Even just smudging every now and again feels positive and lifts my spirits. Using all these therapies and techniques helps to keep me on an even keel, making me feel happy and healthy and putting my relationships in a good place, too.

So, that's the woo-woo out of the way. Now we can look closely at our mental wellbeing and what practices or rituals we can do to keep us balanced.

MENTAL WELLBEING

My mental health started to become an issue in my early forties, which, in hindsight, was the same time that other perimenopause symptoms started appearing. I was prescribed antidepressants, but I knew at the time that it was something more. I wasn't just sad or blue; it was something beyond my control.

George agreed, and was adamant it was something else, because he knew I had it in my nature to be so positive and happy. At the time, I took the antidepressants offered by my doctor, but not for long, because of the effect they had on me, as I mentioned earlier. Now, I know there is a place for antidepressants and some women do need to be on both HRT and antidepressants, because they can happily sit side by side, working together to really help. And it's not a failing to admit that you need help. If you have a broken leg or an infection you would ask an expert for help, and it's the same with your mental health. You mustn't see this as a weakness; if anything, you're stronger for knowing that you need help and are seeking it.

I know the menopause hasn't helped my mental well-being much, but I also think that I'm just pretty worn out from pushing myself from pillar to post and getting myself into situations that have battered me down a bit over the years. It doesn't take much to trigger an anxiety attack when things start to go wrong; I worry much more than I used to and sometimes the negative thoughts just repeat themselves over and over in my head. According to a National Science Foundation study, 95 per cent of our thoughts are repeated and 80 per cent of those thoughts are negative.

Sometimes something I have said or done will just stay with me and I go down the rabbit hole reliving and rehashing it, over and over. Sometimes I just can't shake it off. For me, exercise really helps; when I'm really in a funk and nothing is helping, I suddenly jump to jolt myself out of it. As ridiculous as this sounds, it changes the energy immediately and breaks the bad mood. I do feel silly and realise I must look just a bit odd jumping down the high road when I am out and about with George, but it does the trick, makes me laugh – makes us both laugh – and the mood dissipates.

I guess we all have light and dark sides to our personalities, and we must have both to know when to appreciate the good days. It's all about balance, after all.

For some of us, HRT helps to keep us in line with the four pillars of health I described above and our overall wellbeing. I will caveat that by saying it doesn't just magically make everything perfect again. Life can be challenging, there are struggles and some of those struggles happen daily.

PHYSICAL WELLBEING

Not doing exercise leaves me very low, as I find I now need those happy hormones that are released when I work out, because the endorphins help to relieve stress, flooding my brain with oodles of serotonin. That, for sure, has a positive effect all round.

As I wake early, at around five most mornings, I take advantage of that and get myself out and about either to a class with my PT, a Pilates session or an hour's walk or run around the neighbourhood, taking in that fresh air. Any form of movement never fails to lift my mood, helps to relieve stress and tension and leaves me happier and more able to cope with anything that may come my way. I encourage all of you to pick a fun physical activity – or a few, to keep it varied) – and just stick with it, as it will have an all-round positive effect.

There are other methods to enhance your physical well-being that don't necessarily involve getting hot and sweaty, and most can be done at home.

Body brushing

I've long preached the benefits of body brushing, as it is fantastic for stimulating lymphatic drainage and helping to improve circulation, and it literally takes a couple of minutes. This is a great trick in the summer when the lower half of your legs can become puffy and slightly swollen, but also in the wintertime when skin becomes drier and more dehydrated, when you are maybe eating and drinking more than usual on those dark, chilly evenings and having late nights, especially around festive celebrations.

Body brushing is great for lightly sloughing off dry dead skin, and it leaves your skin tingling. It's so easy, too, especially if you use your body brush on dry skin just before your bath or shower as part of your morning or evening routine. I use gentle, confident upward strokes, sweeping over all areas of the body. I start from the feet, moving up my legs, arms and tummy, always working in the direction of the heart. Don't forget to brush over your lymph nodes, into your groin and into your armpits and breasts.

Cold-water therapy

As chilling as this sounds, the power of cold-water therapy is incredible for us all. A quick burst of cold water over the body boosts immunity, releases endorphins and tones the skin, so I always finish my warm shower or bath with a cold rinse. At first, try for ninety seconds, then as you get used to the shock, work your way up to doing this for longer. I promise it is worth it, as you will literally be buzzing and so full of life and positivity after. Bracing yourself for that cold blast is also incredible for pushing yourself out of your comfort zone, and is strengthening for mental agility, helping you to overcome other more testing challenges, situations or confrontations in day-to-day life. Make sure to focus on your breathing as the water hits you and try to keep calm – don't start panting or panicking. It's how you breathe through it and keep everything calm and zen-like that will help to strengthen you. Think of the Wim Hof method and you'll soon be ready to invest in an ice bath!

Hot-water bath

Back to basics with this one. The simplicity of running a hot bath, adding your choice of oils and bubbles and some Epsom salts a couple of times a week always feels so indulgent and special. The salts in particular help your muscles to relax, relieve any pain in your shoulders and back and are fantastic if you are struggling with perimenopausal and menopausal aches and pains – from frozen shoulders to knee stiffness. They may also alleviate headaches and possibly even hormonal migraines. Light a candle, lock the door and cherish that 'me time'.

Alternative treatments

I'm a real fan of Chinese medicine and therapies for their wisdom in healing the body, mind and soul. Based on thousands of years of ancient teachings, reading the body and helping to heal on an energetic level as well as physical, treatments like acupuncture, which I find amazing for this new phase of life, help me restore balance, to sleep more easily and alleviate some of my hormonal signs and symptoms. Reflexology is another great treatment that I find extremely relaxing, instilling calm and bringing me back into alignment, which contributes to my overall health and wellbeing.

In addition to physical wellbeing, practising meditation through breathwork, mindfulness and gratitude are essential elements of the 360-degree approach to life. For me, the easiest way to get into a clear mindset is through daily breathwork practice.

Breathing techniques

We never get taught to breathe, it just happens naturally from the moment we are born, although sadly, because of life and stress, we get into bad habits, and maybe because we aren't ever taught the correct way to breathe, we take in short, sharp shallow breaths rather than deep, long, calming ones.

We breathe around 22,000 times a day without thinking about it (thankfully, or I would forget!) – our lungs breathing in the air, removing the oxygen, passing it through our bloodstreams and circulating around our tissues and our organs, keeping us alive.

By breathing correctly, we can change the chemistry in our brains, helping to rewire and retrain ourselves to have more clarity, feel calmer, happier and be more positive – all by simply tuning into ourselves, focusing on the breath and slowing everything down.

Discovering new and quite simple breathing techniques has been a big game changer for me; I have learned how to be more in control of my emotions and my feelings, and I can now calm myself down, motivate myself, feel more connected and grounded and help myself switch off either from stressful situations or at night to enable me to sleep. Quite simply, learning correct breathing techniques has truly transformed my life.

I learned how to breathe in 2020 during lockdown, when the world had just shut down and George and I were recovering from Covid. My lungs were not happy, and nor was I, and I had developed a cough. One morning, I was scrolling through my Instagram and a man popped up. I remember so clearly – it was early, and I was still in bed, attempting to get up and start my day, WFH, as we all were at this time. However, rather than scroll right past this stranger, something stopped me. I felt his energy jump out at me through the phone, his kind eyes, and his voice speaking in the calmest Scottish accent. He was playing very cool music and he was talking about breathwork. This man was Stuart Sandeman, author of *Breathe In Breathe Out*.

I had some degree of experience of breathwork from various wellness retreats I had visited over the years, where I was taught to focus on the breath through movement, especially in yoga and meditations. I knew extremely well that powerful connection you may feel within yourself when you focus on nothing more than movement and breathing. The exhilarating sensations you can create within your body are better than any other high you'll ever experience, I promise.

I always say, to quote the Notorious B.I.G., that when it comes to breathwork it's all about getting high on your own supply. That is truly what it is, and we all have the power to feel it. The best news is that it costs nothing, simply a bit of your time.

Anyway, back to that March morning in 2020 when my life changed for ever. As I joined Stuart's online class, I immediately began to feel the effects of a new way of breathing. Slowly, through my daily 25-minute live breathing sessions with Stuart and his communities, I learned to refocus on my breath flow, and with each deep breath I took, I connected with myself.

He showed me and many hundreds of others how to breathe, and through that breathwork how to manifest what we want and how to visualise our futures. He taught us all for free every morning without fail, and a beautiful community formed where we were all there for each other. These techniques turned into powerful tools and we all have them within us.

I can promise you that, as simple as it sounds, by learning how to breathe again and to breathe properly – by tuning into you for even just five minutes a day – you will reset and reframe what you want. You will be happier and healthier, plus your relationship not only with yourself but with others, too, will thrive. It's mind-blowing how incorporating a simple breathwork practice into your life will change it for the better.

On those nights when sleep isn't coming to me for whatever reason – it could be stress, worries, deadlines or the menopause – I tune into my breath and focus on its movement in and out of my body.

To turn off, or at least turn down, the noise in your head, try the following practice. It isn't complicated – everyone can do it and it takes all of four or five minutes.

So, lie on your back, under the sheets (unless you are too hot; I'll leave that to your discretion). Breathe slowly and deeply and consider the following as you are breathing.

Start by noticing the connection between your body and the bed, focus on your back and travel down your body, starting from the way your head is touching the pillow, how soft the pillow is, then move down to your shoulders, focusing on the feeling between your body and the surface you're lying on. Continue to do this all the way down your body, right down to your toes.

Once you have done the back of your body, bring your attention to the front. Focus on the air in the room. How does it feel on your face? Is it cool? Is it warm? Is there a draught? Do you notice the duvet or covers on you? Are they heavy or light? Maybe your arms are resting on your legs – how does that feel? Scan all the way, noticing the different sensations, until you get to your feet and feel the way they are cocooned by the weight and warmth of the covers. This can all take a couple of minutes or so.

Next, in your mind, start to travel down the left side of your body. Notice how your neck is supported and in contact with the pillow, slightly cushioned in. Feel the connection of your shoulder, the heaviness of your left leg touching the mattress again all the way down to your left foot. Then start the whole process again on your right side.

You will be amazed at how that focus of being so in the moment and in tune with how you're feeling can slow down those thoughts and help to relax you. It is the most simple and calming way to switch off from the day. This also works for a midday disco charge-up, particularly if you are in the throes of menopausal warfare or perhaps your HRT hasn't kicked in yet. Try it – find a room, lie down and give yourself ten minutes to recharge.

Another technique to use in times of daily stress and panic is 'if in doubt, breathe it out'. Stuart Sandeman taught me this exercise. Simply breathe in through your nose for five, six or seven counts, hold for a second, then breathe out slowly through your mouth. You will immediately feel a sense of relief and will reconnect with your breath, and your body will slow everything down. It can totally stop any crisis in its tracks, and help to dissolve any stressful situation. Try it!

I also like to use another technique, which is called box breathing (some of you may know it as mountain breath). Simply count your breath in for four, hold for four, out for four, then hold for four. Continue to do this for at least a minute, or longer if it's feeling good. As you get better at this, you can increase the breath count to five, then six and you will feel a sense of space in your head and a calmness in your body that is so peaceful it's almost like nothing else matters. If you are new to breathing exercises, you might find the holding of the breath a little strange. Try to keep the body and mind calm. There is something called 'air hunger', where the body starts to panic, but just try to remain focused on the calmness in your body. There are so many quick and easy breathing techniques that we can dip into, and all are within our capabilities, within our power so that we can change the way we think and feel in just a few breaths. It might seem impossible and something you can't get your head around, but honestly, do this any time you're feeling stressed and you will notice a difference.

EMOTIONAL WELLBEING

By implementing some simple breathing techniques, you have the power to help and heal yourself. Once you have done your breathwork practice, sit in that moment of still, let your breathing go back to a normal rhythm, then you can start to say – either out loud or quietly to yourself – your chosen affirmations.

Affirmations are positive statements that help to push through the negative thoughts that we have about ourselves. They can help to overcome thoughts that come in and out of our minds uninvited, and when they are repeated often enough, we start to believe them. So, start by saying thank you, thank you, thank you for giving yourself this time for you.

Here are a few useful affirmations to kick off with, ones that I love – but knock yourself out, say whatever you want, bring on that abundance of joy and happiness.

- I am kind.
- I am supported.
- I am enough.
- I am confident.
- I am loved.
- I am powerful.
- I am strong.
- I am successful.
- I am happy.
- I am blissful.
- I welcome love into my life.
- I am healthy.
- All I need is within me right now.
- I wake up motivated.
- I am blessed.
- I am fantastic.
- I welcome everything I have ever dreamed of into my life.

The more often you say these statements to yourself or out loud, the more powerful they are.

Another tip when you first open your eyes in the morning, before you reach for your phone, is to try to check in with yourself. Those first waking moments can make or break how you feel going into your day. So immediately scan through the body, giving thanks for your life, that you live to see another day, taking a few big breaths as you do so. Throw your arms straight up, either above you or in front, and have a good stretch, like a cat.

The point is to start the day gently, without bombarding the brain with emails, messages or social media, so go gentle, even if just for those first few minutes after waking up. Doing this can generate a sense of gratitude, of happiness and positivity that can shift any worries or negativity. Give yourself a chance to start the day the right way.

On days when you feel anxious or have had a challenging night's sleep, tell yourself today is going to be a good day. I call this Jedi mind-tricking yourself. And it works. Try it!

Mindfulness

Practising mindfulness helps me to focus more on what my breath is doing, how it is moving around my body and what my needs might be – do I need to slow down? Stop saying yes to everything? Am I doing too much? Am I moving my body? Am I eating well? So many things have the tendency to create that feeling of being overwhelmed. It's important to recognise what they are, then try to be more present. In a world that is so fast-paced and a culture that thrives on go, go, go and multitasking, mindfulness seems like the only way to keep us balanced if burnout threatens.

I am guilty of all of the above, and I have to be mindful of when I am doing too much and pushing too hard. My symptoms are that I become snappy and fraught with anxiety, I feel constantly negative, my sleep is impacted and any time spent with people is a blur because my mind is either elsewhere or I am working on my phone. To change this, I find writing lists of things to do, being more organised and staying away from my phone (easier said than done) really helps. I try to prioritise time with family and with friends and really be in those moments – not thinking about the past, worrying or feeling regretful and not panicking about what's next.

Making time at the end of the day to wind down and switch off helps me to get into a bedtime routine so that my sleep is of better quality. I also try to leave my phone either just outside the bedroom or switched off while charging it by the bed.

Mindfulness can be simply practised through walking outside and taking in your surroundings. This impacts both physical and mental wellbeing. Being in nature not only resets me, it also clears my head and fresh air keeps me oxygenated, but beyond that, noticing the seasons changing, the buds on the trees, listening to the different birds, spotting creatures and butterflies, reminds me how beautiful the world around us is. It brings me back to the here and now, and I am certain it will work for you, too. Next time you are out for a walk or simply going to the shops, pop your phone in a pocket or a bag, lift your head and look up and around you. Notice the sky, the colours, the textures. Can you hear the birds, the trees rustling, the humdrum sounds of everyday activity? These are precious moments of being present and are a perfect example of living mindfully.

THE SKIN WE'RE IN

We are all ageing – it's a fact of life – but we don't have to look or feel our age, and that is something I think we should all have in our minds, to manifest.

I am hugely proactive about embracing ageing as it is so much more positive than being anti-ageing. As I have said before, this is not about choosing to give up and give in, but having a sense of acceptance that things are changing as the years pass and keeping a positive attitude and gratitude for our health. Being pro-ageing is a much more encouraging way to look at the inevitable changes that take place in our faces and bodies, so let's all aim to feel the best we possibly can in our own skin, by looking after it in the best way we can.

Beauty and skincare, for me, have really been a lifelong obsession. It all started at the age of eleven, when I first slipped out the tweezers from my mum's make-up bag and proceeded to pluck my eyebrows to within an inch of their lives. Not a good look for such a young girl, according to my parents. I, however, thought I looked very grown up, and I have to say looking at my passport picture that was taken a few days later, and which I kept for another ten years, I still think I did a brilliant job.

Now, I realise that was the moment I became obsessed with beauty, make-up and skincare.

My Auntie Pepe, a beautiful, elegant Spanish lady, used to work in a department store at the Kanebo counter (a Japanese skincare brand) and she would come home with samples in her handbag and give them to my cousin Ana and me. That fuelled my fire and desire for lotions and potions, firmly cementing my love affair! I also got a facial steamer for my twelfth birthday (although, thinking back, I really didn't need to be steaming my delicate skin, squeezing out imaginary blackheads, rubbing it aggressively with the apricot scrub that I always spent my weekly pocket money on). So, it was clear from an early age that I was destined to work in or with beauty.

I feel incredibly lucky to still have good skin after all I have done to it over the years, and I believe that is in part down to genetics. In addition to scrubbing and steaming, I have subjected my skin to other unnecessary trauma, such as the sun (we overlooked the damage it was causing to our bodies), sugar, alcohol, late nights and partying, lack of sleep and smoking – yes, I know, a disgusting habit, a waste of money and a hideous thing to do to my health, as well as my skin. I have to say that is one of my only regrets in life; I truly wish I had never started, so if you are reading this and are still smoking, if you only do one positive thing for your health, please try to stop.

Sadly, you can't completely reverse the damage from smoking or too much sun exposure, but by stopping smoking, you'll be getting more oxygen and nutrients to the skin, almost instantly looking and feeling better, and immediately there will be less stress on your body, more colour in your cheeks, more energy everywhere. I should also mention that by wearing an SPF you can prevent further skin ageing and pigmentation developing. Add to that a good at-home beauty regime and you will notice an enormous difference to your skin, improving luminosity and texture, as well as tone.

There are lots of treatments available to improve our skin, including lasers to tighten and to resurface, IPL, microneedling and chemical peels, Botox to soften wrinkles and lines, as well as to help prevent further frown lines and, of course, there are fillers. Some of these can be expensive, as well as slightly painful and some are extremely painful (for these a numbing cream is usually applied first to prevent too much discomfort).

I have tried many different beauty treatments over the years, and none of them are cheap. Treatments like microneedling are great for helping the skin to rejuvenate by stimulating it to produce more collagen and skin tissue, in turn smoothing, toning and promoting a healthy glow. Varying needle lengths are used in this procedure; some barely scratch the surface to create a healthy glow and enable products to penetrate, while other more extensive sessions require gas and air and some anaesthetic beforehand. The latter can leave your skin with little scabs and blood. I have never had that type of treatment before, but I know lots of ladies who have had it for acne scarring and are extremely happy with the results. This is a treatment that is less invasive than some others, but even so, you might only do it a couple of times a year to freshen up the complexion.

Fraxel is used for deep lines and sagging. I have witnessed this treatment in action, and it is rather brutal. An anaesthetic is applied that will last for at least an hour, but even then, you do feel pain (how much depends on your pain threshold and how sensitive your skin is). I have had a few other facial lifting treatments, like blue-light therapy – an intense but painless treatment to shock the fibroblasts (connective tissue cells that make collagen) to create new cells and collagen structures with the effect of plumping and supporting the face.

I have also tried thermage, which is a skin-tightening treatment that is safe enough to use around the eyes to help lift baggy eyelids, as well as the lower half of the face to help reduce jowls and fight gravity. Another option is a machine called the ultra-former. I have tried this, too, and even though I took paracetamol, as recommended by the therapist, I wished I'd drunk a hip flask of whisky, it was that painful. But again, this depends on your pain threshold, on how new the machines are or where they are made and, of course, how skilled the therapist is.

For all these treatments it takes up to six months to see the results, and while I have to say they are all fantastic, be warned that they are very expensive and usually need more than one appointment for the desired results, followed by a top-up every couple of years.

I have stayed away from lasers so far, but I do know many people who use them for pigmentation. I personally worry about this method as it is rather extreme and can make the skin thinner, then as soon as you go back in the sun, even with a 50-plus SPF, those dark spots and patches do unfortunately come back.

Profhilo is another option in the form of injections into your face and neck containing hyaluronic acid that helps the skin to produce more collagen, as well as promoting a gorgeous glow. Two treatments are normally required for best results. Another good option is the oxygen facial, which promotes more freshness.

With any of these treatments, a course is recommended, and again they are not cheap, but I see these as preventative in fighting gravity, tightening and lifting the jowl area, the neck and firming around the eyes. The result is a more youthful appearance without the need for a more invasive surgery like a face lift, a half lift or eye surgery. Now, of course, if that's something you want to do as well, there are many options available.

If you are brave enough, there are some amazing surgeons out there who do incredible work, but I don't know if I could do it, so instead I opt for these maintenance treatments – like going to the gym but for our faces. If you have the money and you are deeply unhappy about any part of your face or body, it is 100 per cent your choice what you do, and your happiness and confidence are everything.

Cost is just one of the things to consider before you go ahead. Ask yourself also, are you doing it for you? Will this make you happy? Are there other issues that you think might be the problem? Surgery doesn't equal fulfilment – remember that. If you know that a cosmetic fix is something you *really* want to do, make sure you have properly considered and researched good, reputable surgeons. Then, and only then, go ahead.

The skin is an incredible organ, the largest we have, and it is known as our third kidney, due to the way it can expel toxins. It is living, breathing and protects your body from germs and regulates body temperature. There are many different skin types and so many conditions, so the sooner we get a handle on the skin type we have, the easier it's going to be to manage it in day-to-day life to keep it looking its best.

If you suffer with an oily T-zone, and are more prone to breaking out, then you have combination skin. If you find you are on the more dry and irritated side, most likely you have dry or potentially sensitive skin. Below is a list of skin types and conditions, and I recommend you take the time to find out which you have. Remember, skin types and conditions can change over the years, so pay attention to what yours is telling you.

- Combination
- Dry
- Irritated
- Hormonal
- Rosacea
- Oily
- Open pores
- Blackheads
- Spider veins or thread veins
- Pigmentation
- Melasma

I feel that a healthy glow is what we all aim for as we get older, but unfortunately it gets harder to achieve as the years go by. With menopause, luminosity fades, skin can flare up and become irritated and sensitive and you may find you don't recognise it any more.

Taking care of my skin as I have got older is a big part of my self-care ritual. The way our skin looks can have a huge impact on our confidence. So here are a few simple tips that don't take long at all, and which I swear by. When it comes to looking after your skin, you can keep it simple, but I promise your skin will thank you for a little effort, and you will notice the difference so quickly, so try to stick to these guidelines as much as you can.

CLEANSING

When it comes to your skin, good hygiene is imperative. Cleansing is amazingly simple and quick to do, and will remove all the daily grime, dirt and pollution, as well as any make-up and the residue of creams or SPF – which I hope you are all wearing religiously! (More on that soon.)

Cleansing should be at the top of the list when we talk about skincare. Think of all the dirt you pick up on your hands throughout the day and how often we wash them because of this. Exactly. Well, when dirt, grime, grease and pollutants cling to our skin, this can mean bacteria build up and cause blocked pores, blackheads and acne, and other unpleasant skin conditions will thrive, too.

Now there is a camp of people who seem to find that just giving their face a good old wash with soap and water is enough, and actually my mum is one of those. This baffles me because I don't understand how we could be so different – I'm obsessed with slathering myself with all sorts of concoctions, but my mum loves to keep it simple. I have to say she has got bloody good skin, so genetics must play a huge part.

I suggest choosing cleansers that feel luxurious in texture and are a joy to use. I prefer to use oils, balms and milks to cleanse my face and neck, as they melt away my make-up and are gentle enough to use on my eyes, too. You might prefer a cleanser that you add water to, but make sure they aren't too drying or leave the skin feeling tight. If you are a soap-and-water kind of gal, please take care and look out for signs that your skin is telling you it's unhappy. Soap can sometimes strip the skin too aggressively, which upsets the pH balance and can cause the skin to panic and produce more oil in response.

The ingredients you should be looking for in your skin-care as you get older do change. You want to keep your skin clean, so as not to allow bacteria to cause unsightly breakouts, and you need to know what ingredients are suitable if a bout of hormonal-induced cystic acne does erupt. I use a cleanser with a combination of AHAs (alpha-hydroxy acids), lactic acid and glycolic as well as salicylic acid, which help to alleviate redness and keep my skin clean. Unfortunately, at this time in our lives, some of us might suffer with angry, unsightly spots on our jawlines, chins, up around the ears and on our backs. To keep your skin really clean, incorporate a gentle exfoliant a few times a week to prevent a build-up of blocked pores, bacteria and blackheads.

If you are struggling with extreme breakouts, the first rule is please do not pick, squeeze or pop them, however tempting it may be. This results in scarring, and I mean permanent scars. I learned the hard way and have a few scars to show for it. Avoid touching them, too, as you may also cause them to spread. My top tip? Grab an ice cube from the freezer and apply it to the area to take down the swelling, redness and inflammation, especially if you are on your way out of the door for a big night out or an event. You might want to see a dermatologist if they get really bad, painful or unsightly, but from my experience, it's the hormonal fluctuations that cause these angry flare-ups.

You may see retinoids and retinol listed on products; these are both forms of vitamin A. Beauty gurus swear by this vitamin as an excellent way to encourage skin and cell turnover, resulting in a more youthful, smoother complexion, and it's ideal for tackling scarring and uneven pigmented skin. It also helps with collagen production to increase plumpness and improve fine lines and wrinkles.

The golden rule when cleansing is to always remove your make-up before bed. Be sure to cleanse down to the neck and décolleté (basically, down to the boobs), too, as that is an area that is often neglected. The mistake I made for years was thinking that my skincare regime didn't need to include these areas, but let me warn you – the neck is one of the first places to show your age. This is because it has much less robust skin, with fewer sebaceous glands (naturally producing oil), so it's effectively drier, more delicate and much thinner.

The lower half of my face also started to change dramatically through perimenopausal and menopausal years – not just the firmness, but also the structure started to shift, with muscles sagging along with my jawline. Now that did freak me out. That is why it most definitely requires some love and attention, as well as protection.

New terms like tech neck have popped up here and there because we are often glued to our devices for most of the day, heads bent forwards, looking down. Looking down pulls the face forwards, shortens the muscles in the neck and is not ideal for any of us, especially us women. We want to elongate our necks, lift our faces and jaws, not help gravity by letting it all hang over. So, with the cleansing motion, try to use upward movements to go against that gravitational pull, and throughout the day, try to counteract the posture of looking down by lifting the chin to look at the ceiling, taking breaks to stretch.

DRY AND LACKLUSTRE SKIN

Dry, irritated skin with a lack of luminosity is a major concern for many, and during perimenopause and menopause we find we need to feed and nourish our skin with hydrating and plumping ingredients. Hyaluronic acid is a terrific addition to skincare, helping to boost moisture levels, lessen the appearance of pigmentation caused by sun damage and soften fine lines and wrinkles on the skin.

Always apply these serums on damp skin – so straight after cleansing and before you apply your moisturiser and SPF. Avoid any products with alcohol in them, as these will strip the skin and cause an aggressive reaction.

EATING FOR YOUR SKIN

The experts say that our skin reflects what is going on inside our tummies; some doctors are even able to use different areas on the face to spot whether you are gluten or lactose intolerant. It's so clever that the face can show this, and these areas of congestion reflect your general health.

As we all know, stress plays a massive part in poor skin, and conditions like psoriasis and rosacea can be linked to gut problems. Now when I say this, do not panic – it may just mean your nutrition needs to be looked at for any intolerances, as well as keeping an eye on your digestion. See this as your body giving you a warning sign that something isn't quite right.

As we get older it's a fact that our microbiomes, which live in the small and large intestines, are much more unbalanced. The levels of daily stress and worry take their toll, and with the impact of menopause added to the mix, as well as perhaps years of taking various medications (the contraceptive pill, for example), eating too much of the wrong kinds of food (sugar, alcohol) and bombarding and overloading our systems from time to time, it's no surprise that the way our guts are working is affected. And this, in turn, impacts our skin. This may go on unnoticed for years, but as we start to get older these issues start to show.

Our gut health is so important and not only does it play a huge role in keeping us physically healthy, the microbiome is also responsible for keeping our minds happy (they call the gut our second brain). And the brain has a direct effect on the gut, too, so as we enter perimenopause and menopause that is why so many of us have tummy issues. Whether it is IBS-like symptoms, bloating, constipation or diarrhoea, the decline in oestrogen plays havoc with the entire system, and the gut is hugely affected. To minimise unpleasant symptoms at this stage of our lives, we need to aim for a regular diet that's rich in diversity and all the good stuff.

SKIN AND DIET TOP TIPS

BY RHIANNON LAMBERT (RHITRITION), NUTRITIONIST, AUTHOR AND HOST OF THE *FOOD FOR THOUGHT* PODCAST

As we age, the amount and quality of collagen and hyaluronic acid that our bodies produce decreases, but what's important to remember is that this is totally normal and all part of the ageing process. Here are some of my top nutrition tips for helping to support your skin health.

Remember to eat the rainbow; you may have noticed that many anti-ageing creams or moisturisers contain retinol, a form of vitamin A, which may help improve skin elasticity and the appearance of wrinkles. Retinol also helps with skin cell turnover, which is needed to maintain healthy skin and remove any dead skin you may have. Vitamin-A-rich foods include yellow, red and green leafy vegetables, like spinach, carrots and peppers, as well as eggs, liver and liver products, dairy products and fortified foods.

Don't forget those healthy fats. Fats are often thought of as the enemy, but certain ones, such as omega-3, which is found in oily fish, walnuts, flaxseeds and chia seeds, are beneficial to overall health for a range of reasons, and even for our skin health. Although evidence is very limited, some studies suggest that healthy fats may help protect against sun exposure,[1] as well as indirectly preventing skin-inflammation diseases like acne, due to its anti-inflammatory properties. Be sure to include foods that contain protective antioxidants, such as tomatoes, blueberries, spinach, avocados and garlic.

Your diet may also help with sun protection alongside your usual SPF. Vitamin E is found in some dark green veggies, seafood, nuts and seeds and may be beneficial in reducing UV damage to the skin. Recent research has found that eating almonds, which are a good source of vitamin E, may help to improve your skin's resistance to the sun's rays.[2] Including a handful of these as an on-the-go snack or as a topping on breakfast bowls is one way in which you can help prevent the effects of the sun on your skin health. A good tip here is to make sure you're having food rich in vitamin C, such as kiwis, peppers, oranges and broccoli, as this supports absorption of vitamin E.

To help improve wrinkle severity and skin tone, another recent study[3] on almonds showed that eating these nuts every day had a positive effect on skin health. They found that the appearance of wrinkles was reduced and skin pigmentation improved. However, more research across a larger number and wider range of participants is needed to understand the short- and long-term effects of almond consumption on skin health.

Try to include lycopene-rich foods in your diet. Lycopene is an antioxidant found in foods such as tomatoes (sun-dried tomatoes and tomato purée have the highest levels), guava and watermelon, so try topping dishes with sun-dried tomatoes or add some guava or watermelon chunks to a fruit bowl. There's evidence to suggest that including these sorts of foods in your diet may help to further protect your skin from the sun's UV rays and reduce the incidence of sunburn.[4]

The good news is that you don't need to give up chocolate. Lots of people think that giving up chocolate will help improve their skin health, and while we need to be mindful of the fact that chocolate is a high-fat/high-sugar food, and so should be eaten in moderation, there is no strong scientific evidence to show that eating it causes acne. A lot more scientific research is required; and in fact, there is some evidence to suggest that eating dark chocolate may actually be beneficial to our skin due to its high flavonoid content, which might help with the maintenance and protection of our skin health.[5]

Don't forget to stay hydrated. Water is an essential part of our diets. Most of the body's vital processes need water so that we can function properly, so making sure we get enough is of utmost importance. Including more water in our diets can be as easy as adding in more hydrating foods to our meals; because up to 30 per cent of our daily water intake can come from the food that we eat[6] it's important to include foods with a high-water volume on a daily basis, especially when the weather is hot. (The other 70 per cent comes from drinking plenty of fluids throughout the day. In the UK it is recommended that we consume around eight glasses or 2 litres of water each day.) The most common types of hydrating foods include most fruit and veg, like strawberries, watermelon, peaches, cucumber, lettuce, tomatoes and citrus fruits, as these have a high water volume. These foods also contain lots of essential vitamins and powerful antioxidants for optimal function in the body, in addition to supporting our skin and overall health.

Despite what some 'diet experts' say, you don't need to cut out dairy. Foods like dairy products and high-fat/high-sugar foods have long been demonised by the media for causing skin conditions like acne. The truth is that while there is some evidence that poor diets, particularly those with a high consumption of these foods may cause acne,[7] a lot more scientific research is needed to confirm this, and we need to look at other underlying causes, such as medical conditions and lifestyle choices, not just diet alone. What's great to see, though, is that researchers are looking more and more at how diet may impact skin health, so that in the future we may be able to support our skin with the food we eat alongside a healthy and balanced lifestyle.

OILS

Oil. Such a dirty word, isn't it? It conjures up visions of oil slicks, greasy food, deep-fat fryers and greasy T-zones, so it's no wonder we're wary of slathering it on our faces. But oily fish, olive oil, nuts, seeds and avocado all contain good fats and a high oil content and are known to work wonders for our skin, hair and nails, not to mention the benefits for our minds, joints, metabolism and hormones. So, knowing this, doesn't it make sense to nourish our faces with oils, too?

Quite often, people look at me in horror when I mention facial oils, assuming they leave behind a greasy residue. They worry this build-up will lead to breakouts, but this isn't the case. Depending on the formula, and what other ingredients are in there, oils and essential oils have a healing and calming effect on our skin. In fact, when I went into the *I'm a Celebrity* camp, I was allowed to take my omega oils with me. I was taking them for a hormone imbalance (I was perimenopausal, but I had no idea), but halfway through the show, when my skin was craving moisture, I cracked open a capsule and sneakily massaged the oil into my face! My complexion was instantly soothed and hydrated. I kept at it until I left camp, and no one knew – that can be our little secret!

During the cold winter nights in the UK, I like to hibernate and look after my skin, which has a tendency to become extremely dry in response to the combination of chilly weather and central heating. Sometimes after cleansing my face I like to sit in front of the fire while I am watching TV. I will massage my moisturiser, blended with some delicious smelling oils, into my face in circular, upwards motions. I've now made it my mission to convert others to the healing power of oils. Conditions such as eczema, psoriasis and acne can all benefit from a wisely chosen oil-based treatment; just a few drops on freshly cleansed skin or added into your moisturiser at the start or end of each day can energise your skin and calm a multitude of problems.

These days, a lot of brands are calling their oils 'oil serums', so as not to freak people out. And I get it, I really do – for those of us with oily or combination skin, the idea of adding more oil to our faces seems crazy. However, oils can help to rebalance and correct the overproduction of sebum.

Neroli is a heavenly smelling oil perfect for my dry complexion, but if you have more of a combination skin and need to rebalance excessive oil production, go for a ylang-ylang formula.

If you're oil phobic, I hope this has convinced you to give it a go – I promise your complexion will radiate health!

COLLAGEN

Collagen is responsible for the healing process and the plumpness associated with the skin of our youth, but from around our mid-thirties the body's ability to produce this important protein starts to slow down – we lose the plumpness and then the lines, wrinkles and crows' feet start to become more noticeable – so it's a good idea to try to boost collagen levels, if possible.

You can do this by eating good-quality protein such as fish and fish skin, as well as bone broths and collagen supplements – of which there are many on the market. Most of these contain sugar, which has an adverse effect on the skin, breaking down its structure and attacking the cells, causing more ageing, so always go for a pure collagen product – one that is either marine or bovine – and check that it is sourced ethically and sustainably.

Another good way to encourage the skin to increase collagen production is by using a retinol or by investing in some of the facial treatments I mentioned earlier. With retinols, go slowly, as they increase the skin's turnover and sometimes cause sensitivity and peeling. These products, I feel, are better used in the winter months, unless you go for a lower percentage of retinols, but always remember to apply sunscreen every day (even in the winter months), as your skin can have the tendency to become more sun sensitive. In recent years there has been a boom in the number of products and suncreams on the market. There are two types of UV light: ultraviolet A (UVA), which has a longer wavelength and is associated with skin ageing; and ultraviolet B (UVB), which has a shorter wavelength and is associated with skin burning. When buying suncream, a sun protection factor of at least 30 SPF is advised to protect against UVB, and at least a 4-star UVA protection.

PIGMENTATION

I do now think with some regret how much better my skin could or would have been if I hadn't taken it all for granted. Sugar, alcohol, sun and smoking make a deadly combo, as we all know, because the sun and smoking attack the structure of our skin, breaking down the collagen and causing premature ageing, fine lines and wrinkles, as well as those dark sun spots that start to develop over the years.

I have struggled with pigmentation for the last twenty-odd years, and it is has been the bane of my existence. In my late twenties, I literally had the darkest pigmentation on my upper lip that looked like a moustache, and I was really conscious of it and embarrassed. Every time I so much as looked at the sun this dark shadow would appear and I would try to cover it, but lo and behold, as soon as I glanced at the sun again, it would reappear. No amount of make-up would cover it – or at least I didn't have the skills to do it back then.

All this was entirely my fault because when I used to be on photo shoots as a model I'd be up early and standing in the sun all day with make up on and no SPF, because thirty years ago we were not as aware of the damage caused by the sun or the dangers of being out in it without any kind of protection. Some of the products we used might have had a little bit of SPF – maybe a 15 – but that doesn't really touch the sides as far as giving you ultimate coverage and protection. Added to that, as soon as we broke for lunch, I would be out there by the swimming pool stripped down to my bikini, soaking up as many rays as possible. I would still have the morning's make-up on my face and I knew that in the afternoon I'd be going back into that sun with a light reflector blasting at me, standing in the beating heat of the day.

Having also been on the contraceptive pill – and knowing now that hormones and sun do not mix well together – it doesn't surprise me that ten years later I started to develop pigmentation. This is why a lot of pregnant women develop a 'mask of pregnancy', which is melasma on the face, usually on the forehead, that shows as a big patch of darker pigmented skin. My pigmentation migrated from my upper lip to my forehead. Over the years, I've used different treatments and products to lighten and brighten the area, but in my experience, it just takes a little bit of time to do this, as well as extreme caution in the sun and being vigilant in applying your SPF all year round.

So, to tan or not to tan? For me, it's a no-brainer. While I love how a tan makes me feel – leaner-limbed, braver with the prints and colours I'll wear and more confident when it comes to wearing less make-up – the downsides are just too hard to ignore. Ultimately, I don't want my skin, or my health, to pay the price for a suntan.

But there is another way. For those of us who love a golden, year-round glow, there's the guilt-free alternative in the form of fake tan. We're spoiled for choice when it comes to choosing a product, so here's my guide to achieving bronzed skin from a bottle.

When it comes to choosing the best self-tan, be realistic about how your skin would naturally react in the sun. If you have fair colouring, an intense, dark shade will look more orange than sun-kissed siren. When applying self-tan, preparation is key. Scrubbing the skin before application is preferable because fake tan will develop unevenly on areas of dry skin. Once your entire body is clean and dry, apply pea-sized amounts of moisturiser to your elbows, knees and ankles, along with any other patches of coarse skin. Then begin to apply your chosen product – I like to use a mitt and long, sweeping motions. Once an all-over, even layer is achieved, pay particular attention to your hands. At this stage, use a dry brush to buff around your hands and blend any areas that need it.

Remove any build-up of product from your palms before moisturising your knuckles and nails. This will help to banish any tell-tale signs of a tan applied from the bottle. During the days that follow and to prolong the life of your expertly applied tan, apply a rich, oil-free moisturiser over the top to keep your skin hydrated.

SKIN COMPLAINTS

I've suffered from a skin complaint – more of an annoyance that won't go away – since around the age of ten, in the form of a few scattered bumps on my cheeks. Having always been skin obsessed, I couldn't leave these alone. I wasn't worried – they didn't look like anything sinister, and my mum was also a sufferer (yes, it's hereditary) – but on closer inspection, and when picked(!), I found that these rough, red bumps could be squeezed and they contained a small, hard residue. Or gunk, to put it bluntly!

I got into the bad habit of picking at these marks. While they don't have a head, they certainly do make a satisfying pop. I quickly discovered this made my skin worse – scabbing over and prolonging the life of the lumps, not to mention the broken capillaries and scars caused by all that trauma to my skin.

Fast-forward ten years to my twenties, and the little bumps had spread to my arms. It wasn't until a few years ago, though, that I realised these bumps have a name. After saving my pennies and booking a trip to a pricey dermatologist, I was finally given some answers. The specialist explained I was suffering from keratosis pilaris.

So, what is this exactly? It's basically a condition that affects those of us with dry skin, and it gets worse in the winter months. An overproduction of keratin – a protein – builds up in the hair follicles causing a lumpy, goosebumpy appearance, hence its nickname, chicken skin. It's a common complaint, and after posting about it I couldn't believe the response I received. Men and women of all different ages came forwards to share their KP stories. It turned out I was far from alone in my suffering.

The condition mostly targets the back of the arms, the face and the legs. Over the years, I've tried everything: I have scrubbed, rubbed, exfoliated and buffed. There have been masks and loofahs, retinols and creams. It's safe to say I've spent a small fortune, investing in all sorts of gorgeous, premium creams intended for my face and décolleté. I tried products at much lower price points, too – Epsom bath salts and magnesium. You name it, I've bathed in it. And what's worse, the dermatologist's prescription didn't help my KP either. I was sent away, 'assured' that the condition would clear up in my fifties. I was thirty-six at the time.

So I want to speak frankly about this skin complaint. I want to share my advice on what works and what doesn't. I must be honest, there's no quick fix, but with some dedication and patience you should see some improvement in around six weeks. Stick with it, and I hope, like me, you'll feel and notice a difference – because while my KP hasn't totally gone, I'd say with regular care I'm 90 per cent bump-free. What's helped me the most is moisturising, especially in the winter months when skin tends to be on the drier side. In the summer months, I found it cleared up much more. A combination of using richer and thicker creams with SPF of at least 30, and the sunlight most definitely helped. You can also look into products that contain lactic and alpha hydroxy acid, which stimulate the skin's natural exfoliation and renewal process. But be warned, these can make your skin much more sensitive to sunlight.

COLONICS

It often raises eyebrows when I say I'm a fan, so I wanted to get to the, ahem, bottom of this subject. Before my first experience, over fifteen years ago, I had the same nagging questions as everyone else. What are the benefits? How does it work? Will it hurt?

I had always believed my body did a perfectly excellent job of cleansing itself, without needing the assistance of water and tubes. I assumed colonic irrigations were a fad. After a bit of research, though, I discovered this treatment was anything but new and that Chinese and Indian civilisations, as well as the ancient Egyptians practised colonics.

So I thought I'd get to grips with how the digestive tract works.

For starters, our colons are around 1.5 metres long – that's a whole lot of colon squashed into a small space. It was beginning to make sense that such an intricate system might need a little help now and again. Having always had a sensitive tummy – particularly in times of anxiety and stress – I was starting to come round to the idea of colonics and treating this organ at its source. When I heard the list of conditions that colonics are known to treat – bloating, gas, stress, skin conditions – I knew I had to try it for myself.

And I wasn't disappointed. In fact, it was fascinating how my therapist could assess my digestive health just from examining my poop. Having sought treatment for IBS and low energy levels, my first colonic helped to ease both complaints. I was a convert and have since checked myself in for a treatment twice a year. My tummy always looks flatter afterwards, and I shed a few pounds – not to mention the increase in my energy levels. Colonics also make me more conscious of what I consume, and I now watch out for foods that I know are hard to digest.

I'm always banging on about good gut health. Keeping an abundance of beneficial bacteria in my belly is, for me, the key to feeling good. Admittedly I was a little anxious to hear that colonics strip out everything – the good along with the bad – so after a treatment I would advise taking a course of high-strength probiotics to get the good bacteria back on track. I take probiotics every day anyway, and there are some great brands out there. My advice is to go for the live and active bacteria, and also incorporate what Professor Tim Spector calls the four Ks: kefir, kimchi, kraut and kombucha.

So, what can you expect from your first colonic? The treatment itself lasts between thirty and sixty minutes and while, yes, there's a tube, it's very small and doesn't feel too invasive. My top tip is to take something along with you to read – a magazine always puts me at ease – or music is good, too. There is usually a sensation of needing the loo, but don't worry, this is totally normal. A therapist is also always on hand, so don't be afraid to ask questions – I always ask lots!

After every treatment, I try to take it easy and stick to eating warm cooked food like vegetable soup. Alcohol and spicy foods are not advisable. And while I totally appreciate this treatment isn't for everyone, if you're suffering from bloating or digestive discomfort, I really recommend giving colonics a go.

MOOD FOOD

I can't stress enough how important diet and nutrition are, not just for our skin but for our general wellbeing. Perimenopause and menopause is not a time to be going on strict diets or restricting ourselves too much; however, we do have to tweak a few things.

As we age, our metabolisms slow down and our muscle mass is on the decline, as well as those pesky hormones yo-yoing out of balance, so certain new habits need to be introduced and in some areas a bit of re-education is needed.

Getting the diet right can really help to manage peri-menopausal and menopausal symptoms, in particular mood. There are many reports suggesting that a diet rich in plant-based food has been found to really help flushes, night sweats and some other unpleasant symptoms. It has also been reported that Japanese women don't suffer as much as us in the Western world with symptoms because their diets are rich in omegas, good fibre and lots of phytoestrogens (more on these on page 201).

MOOD, FOOD AND MENOPAUSE

BY EMMA BARDWELL, REGISTERED NUTRITIONIST, HEALTH WRITER AND FOUNDER OF THE M COLLECTIVE

Most people associate the menopause transition with physical symptoms like hot flushes and night sweats, but it's the psychological symptoms that often blindside women.

Low mood, depression, irritability and rage are commonly reported by my clients, as are feelings of low self-esteem, reduced motivation, anxiety, panic attacks, unexplained fear, tearfulness and difficulty coping. Very often, women say they feel joyless, flat and just not like themselves any more. These feelings can be hard to put into words, which is why so many women suffer in silence.

Oestrogen plays a key role in lifting our moods, as it influences serotonin and dopamine. Progesterone is important too, due to the stimulating effects it has on GABA receptors, which help calm anxiety and encourage feelings of contentment. Women with a history of PMS, PMDD or postnatal depression seem to be more likely to experience mood change symptoms during perimenopause and menopause. Although we're not entirely sure why, it would seem logical that these women are more sensitive to hormone fluctuations.

Diet is key

There's no such thing as a menopause-and-mood diet, but a Mediterranean-style way of eating is a good guide. It centres on minimally processed foods, lots of seasonal veg and fruit, lean protein, whole grains, legumes, nuts, seeds, some dairy and healthy fats like olive oil. Interestingly, it was the Mediterranean way of eating that was used in the famous SMILES trial which saw 33 per cent of depressed participants go into remission after twelve weeks of dietary intervention. A reminder to never underestimate the power of food!

The Mediterranean diet is extremely well studied, so we have lots of data on it. Not only is it linked to a lower risk of depression and cognitive decline (and by the way, women on this diet also have 25 per cent lower risk of heart disease and stroke and 50 per cent lower risk of breast cancer, plus fewer hot flushes), but it tastes good, too! It's not particularly restrictive, which is refreshing at a time when there's so much vilification of food, and it also feels doable for most people in the long term.

Lean protein, such as chicken, fish and tofu, is important for regulating blood-glucose levels and, therefore, mood, along with complex carbohydrates like oats and brown rice and healthy fats such as avocados, nuts and seeds. A lot of women I work with aren't getting enough protein at breakfast, which means their blood-sugar levels peak and trough. Poor blood-glucose regulation can make you feel very irritable and on edge. My favourite two-minute protein breakfast is Greek yoghurt (opt for soya if you're vegan), berries and a generous sprinkle of mixed seeds. Eggs, a protein shake or scrambled tofu are also excellent options.

Feed your brain

There are two essential fatty acids – DHA and EPA – that have been linked with improved brain health. They are both types of omega-3 found in oily fish. They're incredibly important when it comes to the brain's structure as they make up the cell membrane that lets good stuff (like nutrients) in and keeps bad stuff (such as toxins) out. If you're not eating a couple of portions of oily fish – think salmon, mackerel, sardines, herring, anchovies, trout – a week, then you may want to think about supplementing with an omega-3 fish or algae oil.

Think before you drink

For optimal mood management, it's wise to minimise alcohol, as it can lead to fluctuations in oestrogen levels and can even impact the effectiveness of HRT. If you're really struggling with irritability, anxiety and depression, I'd advise removing alcohol from your diet altogether. There are lots of non-alcoholic alternatives these days that taste great.

Caffeine has some beneficial properties (polyphenols have been shown to be neuroprotective) but they can also cause some people to feel more anxious and wired and can trigger palpitations. Try keeping a caffeine diary to see if you're sensitive to it, and always try to keep caffeine consumption to mornings only so it doesn't impact your sleep.

Happy gut bugs, happy you

Looking after your gut health is key to managing hormonal and mental health. The gut microbiota – the community of bacteria that resides in your gastro-intestinal tract – has been linked with circulating oestrogen levels and we now think it can significantly influence emotional health.

Ninety per cent of our serotonin is made in the gut lining, and while this doesn't have a direct impact on serotonin levels in the brain (it can't cross the blood–brain barrier), it does seem to have an influence on gut–brain communication. What we do know is that short-chain fatty acids (SCFAs) like butyrate and propionate, which are produced by the bacteria in our guts, can have a direct impact on the production of neurotransmitters like GABA and dopamine, which, in turn, are linked with good mental health.

The single best way to look after your gut bugs is to feed them fibre, because they thrive on it. Think about including all plant foods, not just fruit and vegetables, including whole grains, nuts, seeds, herbs and spices. Diversity is key, although do try to incorporate dark berries and green leafy veg as much as possible, as they're real powerhouses when it comes to brain health. There's also an argument for including some fermented foods like sauerkraut, live yoghurt, kefir and miso, as they contain live probiotics which can help populate our beneficial gut microflora.

Add in, don't take away

Lots of women I talk to are restricting their food intake in some way. Sometimes because they want to lose the much maligned 'meno belly', but often because they've heard something on social media that vilifies a certain food group, such as carbs. An overly stripped-back diet, one that isn't giving you the calories you need to fuel you throughout the day, can leave you feeling very low, fatigued and miserable.

Make sure you're eating an abundance of health-giving foods. Women often find if they're adding in lots of whole foods they don't have so much space (or desire!) for the less healthy ingredients. And please don't fear carbs; they're an important source of fibre and they help with the production of serotonin, our 'happy' neurotransmitter.

Look at your lifestyle

Sleep hygiene is crucial to getting a good night's sleep (see page 274), but it can look different for each of us. The biggest mistake I hear is women scrolling on their phones in bed and not giving themselves enough time to actually wind down after a stressful day.

Exercise and movement have been shown to be hugely beneficial for mental health, and the good news is they don't have to be overly taxing – even a quick walk will help. Movement oxygenates your brain and can help limit the shrinkage that we naturally experience as we age. Yes, brains shrink, but exercise halts this and has even been shown to increase brain volume.

Exercise also increases the production of something called brain-derived neurotrophic factor (BDNF), which has been likened to Miracle-Gro for the brain. Low levels of BDNF have been linked with depression, as well as certain brain-related disorders such as Parkinson's. Just thirty minutes of aerobic exercise a day can increase BDNF by 30 per cent.

Other factors to potentially add to your toolkit include getting outside in nature, yoga, aromatherapy, massage, CBT, spending time with people who bring you joy, breathwork, mindfulness, guided meditation, journalling, cold-water swimming, acupuncture and reflexology. Ultimately, you need to find what works for you and then make sure you do it consistently.

Think about HRT

Hormone replacement therapy (HRT) may be effective for psychological symptoms and low mood in menopause. Some women report feeling calmer and on a more even keel when they take it. If you can't – or don't want to – use HRT, there are other medications you can discuss with your GP, including SSRIs (antidepressants), which can be taken on their own or in tandem with HRT.

Think about your vagus nerve

Your vagus nerve runs from your brainstem, down through your diaphragm and into your gut. It appears to have lots of roles and is constantly relaying information back and forth between your body and brain. It is thought that 'stimulating' the vagus nerve may have anti-inflammatory and calming effects on the body, in turn helping with things like mood and depression. How can you stimulate it? Singing, chanting, humming, deep breathing ... even cold-water exposure has been shown in some studies to help.

Talk it out

It's important to be able to talk to friends or family at this time. There are also online forums and groups that many women find helpful. Talking therapy, CBT or counselling can be a brilliant adjunct to all of the above (or in its own right) and some women find a life coach useful, especially if they feel they're lacking purpose or suffering low self-esteem and loss of identity.

And finally

Women notoriously have a lot on their plates. Say no to things you don't want to do, don't overcommit yourself, and set boundaries to make sure other people don't encroach on your time. Be bold!

Speaking of time, it's super important to make sure you set some aside for yourself, so I often encourage women to weave short pockets of 'alone time' into their day. Self-care isn't selfish – it's crucial for your wellbeing and so few of us are actually prioritising this for ourselves. Menopause is a time when you really need to take stock of your health and start putting your own needs first.

What's the deal with phytoestrogens?

Phytoestrogens are plant compounds that have mild oestrogen-like properties. The two most-researched types are isoflavones, usually found in soy products, and lignans, commonly found in seeds, legumes and whole grains.

Phytoestrogens work in the body like a weak form of oestrogen. Although much more research is needed to understand them properly, they appear to bind to oestrogen receptors, upregulating some and blocking others.

Foods such as tofu, edamame beans, ground flaxseeds and legumes may help reduce the severity and frequency of hot flushes for some, but not all, women. The research is mixed, but there may well be benefits to eating two to three servings of phytoestrogen foods daily to reduce the frequency and severity of hot flushes. (One serving = 80g edamame beans, 100g tofu or tempeh, 250ml soya milk or 200ml soya yoghurt.)

Combining phytoestrogens as part of a diet rich in plant-based foods seems to provide the most benefits. In one study, when women ate 86g cooked edamame beans daily, hot flushes decreased by 79 per cent. Don't expect overnight miracles, though – it can take two to three months for the benefits of plant oestrogens to be seen and effects can vary between individuals.

There's a lot to be said for plant-centric diets in general when it comes to menopause and vasomotor symptoms. A study of more than 17,000 menopausal women found those who ate more fruit and vegetables experienced a 19 per cent reduction in hot flushes and night sweats. It's also worth bearing in mind that diets rich in colourful plant foods can help lower your risk of chronic diseases such as heart disease, obesity, high blood pressure, diabetes and some cancers – many of which we can become more susceptible to as the protective effects of our hormones decline.

Perhaps the most beneficial aspect of eating plant-based foods is that they provide essential food for your microbiota. As we've already discussed, good gut health is vital at this time of life, not just for digestion, but also for immunity, hormone production and mood. Incidentally, the reason we think phytoestrogens work for some women but not others might be down to a certain gut microbe that converts the soya isoflavone known as daidzein to a more potent form called equol. Interestingly, about 50 per cent of women in Asia are 'equol producers' compared to only 25 per cent in the US. This might possibly be one reason why Asian women report fewer vasomotor symptoms than Western women.

Phytoestrogens also have lots of other nutritional benefits, including protein, fibre, B vitamins and minerals like potassium and magnesium. Soya protein – found in things like tofu, tempeh and edamame beans – may also help to lower LDL (sometimes referred to as 'bad') cholesterol. Some studies have additionally shown that phytoestrogens might be beneficial for cardiovascular health, bone density and other menopausal symptoms. One thing to note is that we're talking about minimally processed soya products here, not plant burgers and sausages that tend to be high in salt and fat. I advise seeking out organic and/or non-GMO products where possible.

Does soya increase breast-cancer risk?

Lots of people worry that eating soya will increase their risk of breast cancer. There have been many large-scale studies carried out showing that isoflavones are chemically different to oestrogen and that soya products are safe to eat as part of a healthy balanced diet without increased breast-cancer risk. In fact, some studies link a lower risk of recurrence in women who've had breast cancer and regularly consume soya. A 2017 editorial article in *Cancer* – the official journal of the American Cancer Society – concluded that 'The totality of the evidence suggests that increased soy food consumption decreases the risk of breast cancer and results in better treatment outcomes in both Western and Asian women'. As always, check with your oncology team before making changes to your diet (including starting new supplements).

Soya and thyroid health

There are lots of conflicting messages online about soya interfering with thyroid hormone production. As always, there's a grain of truth that often gets embellished. If you take medication for a hypothyroid disorder (such as Hashimoto's disease), you must leave at least one hour between taking the medication and eating soya. This is because soya can affect the absorption of the medication. It's also recommended that people with low iodine avoid soya until their levels are replete again.

Isoflavone supplements

You can buy concentrated forms of phytoestrogens in supplement form. Common ones are sage, black cohosh and red clover. These haven't been studied in women who have a history of hormone-sensitive cancer or who are taking tamoxifen and so aren't recommended or should only be taken under medical supervision.

An at-a-glance list of phytoestrogens and their sources:

- **ISOFLAVONES:** tofu, tempeh, soya yoghurt, miso, natto, edamame beans, chickpeas, lentils, peas
- **LIGNANS:** flaxseeds (sometimes called linseeds), sesame seeds, cashews, kale, broccoli, Brussels sprouts, carrots, cabbage, cauliflower, peppers, cherries, strawberries, garlic, apples, apricots
- **COUMESTANS:** split peas, pinto beans, lima beans, alfalfa sprouts, red clover
- **STILBENE:** peanuts, grapes

And some foods containing phytoestrogens:

- Soya beans and soya products
- Flaxseeds

- Sesame seeds
- Oats
- Barley
- Beans
- Lentils
- Yams
- Rice
- Mung beans
- Apples
- Carrots
- Pomegranates
- Mint
- Spinach
- Oily fish – omega-3 fatty acids are a group of essential fats that you must obtain through your diet because your body can't produce them on its own
- Dark chocolate – packed full of iron and antioxidants
- Fermented foods – kimchi, kraut, kombucha, kefir, miso, tempeh, as well as live yoghurt for the gut microbiome

CREATING A DIET THAT WORKS FOR YOU

I notice a huge difference in both my energy and my body, depending on what I eat. Sadly, we live in a world obsessed with weight, scales and fad diets, and this can have a big impact on our energy levels and the quality and luminosity of our complexion. I know how important it is to eat well for optimum health, and that eating well is about focusing on a diet rich in variety. Of course, with such a huge range of nutritious foods available, you can always find something that you like that will keep you healthy, but here's what I have found works for me.

We're encouraged to eat five portions of fruit and veg a day, but I think we can consume much more. Think of your plate as a rainbow of foods and know that the more colour you incorporate, the better. I eat as many colourful and water-rich foods as possible, including pomegranates, cucumber, asparagus, kale, spinach, cauliflower, radishes, beetroot and peppers (any colour). All of these are rich in antioxidants and help your skin by preventing or slowing down cell damage.

In total, you should try to include around thirty different plant-type foods into your diet each week. Remember nuts, seeds and pulses all count, as well as all the different herbs and spices, so throw them all into your food, as they not only give it good flavour, but also help to keep your gut healthy, healing you from within.

I always start the day with a hot/warm water with lemon. This is a fantastic way to wake the body up and flush the system through; in short, it gives the body an internal massage, which is great for the organs. I often make myself a healthy juice using ginger, celery, carrots, beetroot and lemon, or blitz up an almond-milk smoothie with blueberries, half a banana and a handful of gluten-free oats.

Good fats such as avocados, nuts, seeds and olive oil are amazing at moisturising the skin from the inside and are good for you and your complexion (in moderation, of course). Protein-rich foods are also important for the production of collagen, so I make sure I include eggs, salmon and lean meats, but I do try to avoid refined carbs most of the week – I swap out white rice for brown, or quinoa, which is more protein than carbohydrate. As much as I adore them, I swap out potatoes for sweet potatoes or squash, and I limit indulging my potato cravings to once a week. It's the same with pasta, pizza and bread. I don't completely take these foods out of my life, as some of them are my ultimate comfort-food favourites – especially pizza, cheesy spuds and a big steaming bowl of pasta – I just know I can't have them as often as I used to. So again, it's about moderation and being sensible, but also allowing myself a treat every now and again.

And don't forget the power of water – it energises the cells in our bodies, helps with digestion and flushes out toxins and fats from our systems. I aim for a couple of litres of water a day, and when I'm feeling tired, I reach for a big glass of H2O to perk me up instead of endless cups of coffee.

I would also like to suggest adopting a new way of looking at eating – intuitively. Basically, this means eating when we are hungry, rather than out of habit or routine. Portions also have to be a little smaller in order to assist a flagging metabolism. A couple of times a week I like to do a fast, leaving a gap of twelve hours – I usually just skip breakfast a few times a week with my first meal being lunch around 12.30/1pm. This is NOT a way of starving myself or trying to control weight; it's just about giving my digestion a rest from constantly having to break down food, which is quite tiring for the body (see page 99). One thing you must promise me is that you will make sure your first meal contains protein and lots of vegetables and isn't a snack but a proper healthy meal.

I avoid snacking as much as possible and concentrate on having three good meals a day packed full of goodness to keep me satisfied for longer and less likely to want to reach for the chocolate mid-afternoon. If I really get a craving, I find that an apple or a couple of dates with a spoonful of almond butter make a yummy treat or, failing that, a square or two of dark chocolate – which is actually quite good for us, being full of iron as well as antioxidants.

Being organised really helps me to stick to a healthy eating programme. I like to write a list or a menu of what the week looks like, and when I get the time, I do some batch cooking, so there is always food ready to grab or take with me on the road to the television studio or on shoots. This way, I know that what I am eating will be healthy and nutritious. This is much easier than you think and just requires a little planning – making overnight oats, or chia seed pudding the night before, or when cooking fish or chicken, I just make extra portions. I also like to roast or steam vegetables, which can be used to make soups, too, and it's also a great way to use up stray veg at the bottom of the fridge.

You can store most of your leftovers or batch food in the fridge for around four days, or even pop them in the freezer in portions. I also like to make turkey chilli (see page 228) – this is delicious, nutritious, low-fat and so easy to make, and you can have it on its own or with brown rice or quinoa. I like to add lots of fresh coriander and avocado on top for extra goodness.

COOKING AT HOME

The key to healthy, nutritious meals is to cook as much as you can at home using fresh ingredients, preferably organic or from a good supplier – either farm shops or your local butcher and fishmonger. Also, try to think about *how* you cook your food – are you always pan-frying? How about steaming your vegetables or roasting your veg or meat?

A well-stocked kitchen means you always have something on hand to cook. I try to have a piece or two of lean animal protein and tins of beans and pulses in my cupboard – chickpeas, kidney and butter beans, as well as lentils – and I always have fresh herbs in the fridge and a fully stocked spice shelf – this means I can always add so much flavour as well as goodness to my cooking.

My ultimate spice selection is ground cumin, turmeric powder, garam masala, ground cinnamon, chilli flakes, ground ginger and paprika. I also like to keep a store of nuts and seeds, including flaxseeds, almonds (raw and unsalted), pistachios, chia seeds, sunflower and pumpkin seeds and pine nuts. These are fantastic to add to your morning yoghurt and fruit as well as your smoothies or overnight oats. I also use lots of nuts in my main courses because they add a vital source of protein and good fats, as well as texture and crunch to dishes. Try toasting them in a dry pan for a few minutes to add more taste and texture.

I love my kitchen-cupboard staples, but when I'm cooking, I don't get too caught up with having all the right ingredients; I say improvise, going with what you have in your fridge and cupboards.

So, I'm going to share a few of my favourite recipes here. Some would say that breakfast is the most important meal of the day, but as I have got older, I do like to fast for longer periods of time, so, as I've mentioned, I sometimes forgo an early breakfast. On these days, I usually opt for my hot water with lemon and then take a black coffee with me to work out. Then, later in the morning I may break my fast with a smoothie or a bowl of fruit yoghurt and seeds or a serving of overnight oats. Some days, I go for eggs, which are an excellent source of protein and there are so many ways to eat them, so you never get bored with them!

So, let's start with some breakfast recipe ideas.

BREAKFAST

BLUEBERRY AND OAT SMOOTHIE

You can add protein powders or collagen powders and take this with you to work or the gym to enjoy for breakfast or as an elevenses snack.

   A handful of blueberries
   ½ banana
   125ml almond milk (or milk of your choice – goat's milk
      is delicious)
   40g oats

This is so simple. Just add everything to a blender and blitz!

BANANA CADO

I love this smoothie; it's rich and chocolatey, and it makes a good substitute for a coffee, as it's the perfect mid-morning pick-me-up.

½–1 banana
¼ or ½ avocado (this adds a creaminess), stoned
1 tsp cacao powder
200ml almond milk (or milk of your choice)

Add everything to a blender with a few ice cubes and blitz.

OVERNIGHT OATS WITH GRATED APPLE, CINNAMON AND SEEDS

This recipe is so easy and everyone loves it. Plus, you can prepare it ahead of time and leave it in the fridge.

2 heaped tbsp goat's milk or yoghurt (ideally sugar-free)

80g oats (I use gluten-free)

1–2 apples, grated

1 tsp ground cinnamon (or to taste)

½ tsp chia seeds

½ tsp pumpkin seeds

1–2 scoops collagen powder (optional)

Combine the milk and oats in a bowl, then stir in the grated apple – as much as you like. Sprinkle over a generous amount of cinnamon and mix, then stir through the chia and pumpkin seeds and collagen powder, if using. Cover the bowl and place in the fridge overnight.

In the morning, simply serve as is or add a handful of berries. It's a yummy, nutritious pre-made breakfast.

EGGS – EVERY WAY

Eggs make a good low-fat, high-protein option to fill you up and act as either a hearty breakfast or a brunch for any day of the week. You can eat them in so many different ways; either boil them (if you make extra, you can keep them in the fridge, so you always have a snack on hand) or scramble them, adding spinach, mushrooms and any other vegetables you have. You can also make an omelette with spinach, onions, mushrooms, peppers and a little hot sauce to add some spice. Always season with salt and pepper – I like to add dried chilli flakes, too.

If you need some kind of bread, I love to heat up a seeded tortilla wrap in a dry frying pan, then throw in the scrambled eggs for a Mexican take, or you can have it on the side. Failing that, a little sourdough slice won't be too bad – just remember: stick to smaller portions.

OTHER EASY BREAKFAST SUGGESTIONS

I sometimes eat fish in the morning, which shocks a lot of people (although people eat smoked salmon with scrambled eggs as a breakfast treat, so I don't understand why it seems so strange to so many). The Japanese eat fish for breakfast with miso soup and vegetables, and as I have mentioned before, that is one of my favourite breakfasts.

I also like a good dollop of yoghurt with some sliced kiwi (high in vitamin C and packed full of fibre) or a bowl of fresh berries with a good sprinkling of nuts and seeds. A delicious way to start the day – easy and so quick.

SOUPS

Soups are so easy to make, and you can pack so much goodness into them, too. Pure health in a bowl. They also keep in the fridge for around three days, so make up a good batch at the start of the week and that way you have something nutritious that you can heat up to eat at any time of the day, or take with you to work.

GARLIC SOUP

This recipe is from my friends Stuart and Nova, and it is rather special.

Garlic soup for health and immunity … I am not going to lie, this is punchy, but it tastes so good and is pure health in a bowl. You might want to avoid people for a day or two after eating it, as the garlic must ooze out of every pore. This will serve four.

26 garlic cloves (unpeeled)
2 tbsp olive oil
2 tbsp vegan butter
1 large onion, sliced
1½ tsp fresh thyme
50g fresh ginger, peeled and finely chopped
½ tsp cayenne pepper
26 garlic cloves, peeled
800ml organic vegetable broth
300ml coconut milk
Sea salt and black pepper

Preheat the oven to 180°C/350°F. Place the unpeeled garlic cloves in a small glass baking dish. Add the olive oil, sprinkle with sea salt and toss to coat. Cover the baking dish tightly with foil and bake for about 45 minutes until the garlic is golden brown and tender. Allow to cool.

When cool enough to handle, squeeze the garlic between your fingertips to release the cloves. Transfer to a small bowl.

Melt the butter in a heavy large saucepan over a medium-high heat. Add the onion, thyme, ginger and cayenne pepper and cook for about 6 minutes until the onions are translucent. Add the roasted garlic cloves plus the raw peeled garlic cloves and cook for 3 minutes.

Add the vegetable broth, cover and simmer for about 20 minutes until the garlic is very tender. Working in batches, purée the soup in a blender until smooth, or in the saucepan using a hand blender.

Return the soup to the saucepan, add coconut milk and bring to a simmer. Season with sea salt and pepper to taste.

HEARTY AND WHOLESOME MINESTRONE

I love a minestrone, and the good news is you can pretty much use whatever you have in your fridge and cupboards for this. I haven't specified amounts here for most of the ingredients, as this is a great one for freestyling – you will surprise yourself. This soup keeps well in the fridge, and is packed full of colourful, delicious vegetables and that all-important protein and fibre, too.

Onions

Celery

Garlic

Carrots

Kale (if you have it, or courgettes)

Olive oil, for frying

1 bay leaf

Sprig of fresh thyme

1 x 400g tin chickpeas or borlotti beans

Chicken stock or water

Tomato purée (optional)

Small pasta, rice or quinoa (optional)

Sea salt and black pepper

Chop up all the veg and add to a pan with some olive oil (just a little).

Season with salt and pepper and cook until the veg have softened. Then add the bay leaf and thyme and chuck in the chickpeas or borlotti beans (fibre and protein, tick!).

Then add in enough chicken stock or water to cover your ingredients. You can add tomato purée if you have some, for more colour and a boost of flavour. And traditionally, minestrone has pasta in it, so add some if you really want it, or use quinoa or brown rice – both great alternatives.

This is literally your soup done. It will need time for the flavours to really enrich, though, so leave it simmering over a low heat for around 30–45 minutes.

RED SPLIT LENTIL SOUP WITH INDIAN SPICES

One of my favourite soups and it's budget-friendly and filling, too. It's so yummy and healthy, packed full of flavour and that all-important protein – and the lentils contain calcium, fibre and iron.

    Extra virgin olive oil, for frying
    3–4 large carrots, diced
    1–2 garlic cloves
    1–2 heaped tsp each of ground cumin, ginger and
        garam masala
    190g red split lentils, rinsed
    Vegetable or chicken stock cube (optional)

Heat the oil in a large saucepan or a deep frying pan, then add the carrots and the garlic, and slowly cook until the carrots start to caramelise a little – I add a splash of water if it looks like it needs it. Sprinkle over the cumin, ginger and garam masala to add warmth and more depth to the soup.

Add the lentils to the pan and stir to coat them in the carrot and garlic mixture. Pour in warm water to cover the lentils, then let it all simmer for 20 minutes, slowly adding more water as the lentils absorb it. If you want to crumble in a vegetable or chicken stock cube you can do, or instead of water you can add a chicken bone broth.

SEXY UP YOUR SALADS

A salad needn't be bland or unappealing and it doesn't have to be cold either; I know on winter days and nights a warm salad with cooked vegetables is something I crave. I also like to add some protein – whether it's beans or pulses, tofu, cheese or lean meats and fish. Pack it full of your favourite ingredients, such as sweet potato (high in the antioxidant beta-carotene, which converts to vitamin A), red quinoa (a gluten-free protein full of vitamins and amino acids) and leafy greens, such as kale (a fibre that will help keep you fuller for longer). As the seasons start to change, we need to feed our bodies with as many colourful food groups packed full of the necessary goodness as possible to protect us from the numerous bugs and germs that take their toll on our busy lives. But along with these main ingredients, I've tracked down some extra magic that we should all be sprinkling in and on our salads to help us feel sexy into the colder months. Get ready to stock up your kitchen cupboards for the ultimate health and sex-life boost!

- **PUMPKIN SEEDS AND OIL:** Try dressing your salads with pumpkin oil (note that due to its low smoke point it's not suitable for cooking). Its nutty sweetness is not only yummy but is known to promote health from the inside out. With one of the highest concentrations of polyunsaturated fats, pumpkin oil can help to lower blood pressure and cholesterol. And its fatty acids and vitamin E promote the growth of new cells, which is great when it comes to hair, skin and nails. Regular consumption has also been shown to help relieve depression and anxiety, lowering stress hormones in our bodies and increasing libido (I love toasted pumpkin oil). For added crunch, why not sprinkle some seeds on top of the salad, too?

- **ZINC:** This super mineral works wonders for our bodies. It helps support our immune systems and kickstarts our ability to metabolise food. Give your salads a zinc boost with garlic – I like mine roasted in its skin – or sprinkle over some sesame seeds for instant added nutrition. Some studies have also shown a link between depression and low zinc levels, so there's even more reason to make sure you're not lacking.

- **FLAXSEEDS:** These seeds are packed full of omega-3 fatty acids and provide an excellent dose of fibre, too. Sprinkle them either roasted or raw on top of your salads for a powerful antioxidant boost. And for you all veggies and vegans out there, flaxseed is a great source of plant-based protein.

- **SALAD SPRINKLES:** If you're looking for a quick
  and convenient addition, many supermarkets and
  health-food stores stock ready-to-sprinkle seed mixes
  for added crunch and flavour.

MEXICAN SALAD WITH HALLOUMI, AVOCADO AND SALSA

I adore this salad; it is so tasty and, again, so simple.
Change it up and add some beans instead of your animal
protein (kidney beans are delicious, too). Or if you want
to make this plant-based, this salad works well with tofu
(the salsa and chilli add a good flavour to what can
otherwise be a rather bland food, although it is an
extremely good source of protein).

1 avocado
1 spring onion, finely chopped
1 baby gem lettuce, roughly chopped
Pinch of dried chilli flakes
A handful of chopped, cooked halloumi, cooked
   chicken breast or tofu cubes
185g cooked quinoa or brown rice

For the salsa

A packet of tomatoes (any kind), chopped

½ red onion, finely diced

A handful of coriander, chopped (optional)

Extra virgin olive oil, for drizzling

1 lemon or lime

Sea salt and black pepper

Start by making the salsa. Combine the tomatoes, red onion and coriander in a bowl. Coriander is zingy and punchy and not everyone's cup of tea, so leave it out if it's not your thing. Season with sea salt and pepper, a splash of extra virgin olive oil and a squeeze of either lemon or lime juice.

Mash up your avocado with a fork to make a guacamole or, if you like it super smooth, you can blend it – I personally like some texture. Combine with the spring onion and baby gem and sprinkle with salt and dried chilli flakes.

Add to a bowl with the halloumi, chicken or tofu and the quinoa or rice – you can add a drizzle of oil over it all and a little more lime or lemon juice, as well as some zest to make it sing even more.

WARM RICE OR QUINOA SALAD

This is great as a main course for four, with any type of
protein, or in the summer with barbecued lamb, chicken,
a piece of salmon or mackerel or some feta. I like to
make a large bowl to accompany a BBQ, along with other
salads, and serve this for the whole family.

185g brown rice or quinoa
½ cucumber, chopped into little cubes
2–3 spring onions, finely sliced
A handful each of parsley, coriander and mint, chopped
Seeds of 1 pomegranate
25–50g toasted pistachio nuts

To serve
Lemon juice
Olive oil, for drizzling
Sea salt and black pepper

Cook the rice or quinoa according to the packet
instructions. Drain and leave to cool for 5 minutes. Tip
into a bowl and stir in all the remaining ingredients. Add
a squeeze of lemon, a drizzle of olive oil and season with
salt and pepper. And there you have it – a yummy,
healthy, warm rice salad.

MAINS

These next two recipes are staples for George and me.

SPICED SWEET POTATOES AND CHICKPEAS WITH A BUTTERBEAN DIP

I love this recipe – it's plant-based goodness at its best. I like to use lots of spices to add flavour. This serves two with a yummy, creamy dip as a side dish, or you can eat it with carrots or any other crudités.

    2 large sweet potatoes, cut into halves then into
        quarters
    Olive oil
    1 x 400g tin organic chickpeas, rinsed and drained
    1 tsp garam masala
    1 tsp ground cumin
    1 tsp turmeric
    1 tsp ground coriander
    Raw spinach or steamed kale, to serve

For the butterbean dip

1 x 400g tin organic butterbeans or cannellini beans,
   rinsed and drained

3 garlic cloves

1 tbsp olive oil

1 tsp garam masala

1 tsp ground cumin

1 tsp turmeric

1 tsp ground coriander

Lemon juice, to taste

Sea salt and black pepper

Preheat the oven to 180°C/350°F.

Add the sweet potatoes to a roasting tin with some olive oil and roast in the oven for 30 minutes.

While the potatoes are roasting, add the butterbeans to a blender, then add the garlic – all or just some, depending on your preference (we like it punchy!). Add the olive oil, spices and lemon juice and season with salt and pepper. Blitz to a smooth texture, ensuring all the garlic has been worked into the mixture.

When the 30 minutes' roasting are up, add your chickpeas to the sweet potatoes with a little olive oil and the spices. This dish can take a lot of spice! Continue to cook for another 35 minutes, giving it a stir halfway through. Serve on a bed of raw spinach or steamed kale.

TURKEY CHILLI

Another dish we have regularly is this version of a chilli con carne, cooked with low-fat, protein-packed turkey mince instead of beef. As with all my recipes, feel free to add or take away anything – I cook very instinctively and don't usually follow a recipe. You can eat this on its own or with some quinoa or brown rice. Always garnish the chilli with fresh coriander, and, for an added Mexican touch, some diced avocado. This is great as leftovers, as it tastes even better the next day, either WFH or if you take it with you to work.

½ onion, red or white, chopped

1 red chilli, chopped

Extra virgin olive oil, for frying

4 garlic cloves

500g turkey mince (if you prefer, use lamb, beef or a combination)

2 x 400g tins chopped tomatoes

2 x 400g tins red kidney beans (I like to use the ones in chilli sauce, as they add an extra kick)

Red wine, to taste (optional)

Bag of fresh spinach (optional)

Throw the onion and chilli into a pan with a little extra virgin olive oil. Add the garlic and cook slowly, until softened. Add the mince, stirring to break it down, until browned, then add the tomatoes and beans. Add the red wine, if using – it doesn't need it, but if you have some left from the night before, chuck it in. Simmer for 1 hour.

After an hour or so of cooking, I add a bag of fresh spinach and leave it to wilt for a minute. Then it's ready to serve!

SLOW-ROASTED SPICY TOMATOES WITH TOASTED ALMONDS

I like to add some cinnamon to this, which is lovely in combination with the tomatoes.

A selection of tomatoes, left whole if small or cut into
    quarters if large
Olive oil, for drizzling
Pinch of chilli flakes
Flaked almonds
185g quinoa
Sea salt and pepper

Preheat the oven to 120°C/250°F.

Start by slow-roasting the tomatoes on a baking tray for 2 hours in the oven. After half an hour, drizzle them with a little olive oil and season with chilli flakes and salt and pepper. I like to add some cinnamon too.

Toast the almonds in a dry frying pan and set aside to cool.

Rinse the quinoa in cold water, then add to a pan with a small amount of water and simmer for 13–15 minutes, or until your quinoa is cooked (light and fluffy).

Add the hot tomatoes to the quinoa and mix it all together, then serve sprinkled with the toasted almonds.

GRILLED SALMON IN GINGER SAUCE

Another recipe that I make more by instinct than instructions! These salmon skewers with ginger, soy sauce and garlic are so easy to make. And it works really well with chicken breast, too. Serve with sautéed mushrooms and steamed kale and a little brown rice. If you like, you can add a couple of eggs to your rice and vegetables – it's delicious!

    2 salmon fillets, skinned and chopped into chunks
    1 tbsp light soy sauce
    Grated fresh ginger
    1–3 garlic cloves, crushed

Simply marinate the salmon chunks in a bowl with the soy sauce, grated ginger and crushed garlic and chill in the fridge for half an hour. Thread the marinated salmon chunks on to metal skewers (or wooden ones that have been soaked in water for half an hour) and grill on a medium heat or a barbecue grill for 8 minutes, turning regularly.

SIDES AND SNACKS

ROASTED BROCCOLI WITH CHILLI AND ALMONDS

I love this broccoli roasted in the oven, drizzled with a little olive oil, crushed chilli and sliced almonds – it makes an amazing side dish.

    1 head of broccoli, cut into slices, lengthways
    Olive oil, for roasting
    Pinch of chilli flakes
    A handful of sliced almonds
    Sea salt

Preheat the oven to 180°C/350°F.

Add the broccoli slices to a baking tray and toss with olive oil, then sprinkle with sea salt and chilli flakes. Cook for 25 minutes, turning once.

While the broccoli cooks, toast the flaked almonds in a dry frying pan.

Once the broccoli has finished cooking, sprinkle with the toasted almonds and serve immediately.

BANANA AND OAT COOKIES

I made this recently after discovering all my bananas had gone black. I didn't want to make banana bread (I think we have all overdone that one!), so I took my overripe bananas and made these instead.

4 overripe bananas
80g gluten-free oats
2 tbsp chia seeds
2 tbsp flaked almonds
A handful dark chocolate chunks or dried fruit
  (optional)

Preheat the oven to 200°C/400°F.

Add the bananas to a mixing bowl and mash them using a fork. Add the oats, chia seeds and flaked almonds and stir to combine, then stir in some dark chocolate chunks or dried fruit, if you like. Bring the mixture together and drop tablespoons of it on to a baking tray lined with baking parchment.

Cook for 25 minutes until lightly golden. So good with a cuppa!

ROASTED CAULIFLOWER WITH TAHINI SAUCE AND POMEGRANATE

This is a real crowd pleaser in my home.

1 head of cauliflower, cut into large florets
3 tbsp extra virgin olive oil
1½ tsp paprika
Sea salt and black pepper

For the tahini sauce
1 garlic clove, crushed
Juice of ½ lemon
3 tbsp light tahini
2 heaped tbsp Greek yoghurt

To garnish
Pomegranate seeds
A handful of mint leaves, finely chopped
A handful of parsley leaves, finely chopped

Preheat the oven to 220°C/425°F.

Throw the cauliflower florets into a bowl, toss with all
the other ingredients and season with salt and pepper,
coating the cauliflower evenly. Transfer to a baking tray,
making sure the florets are evenly spread out. Cook in the
oven for 40–45 minutes, turning halfway.

Meanwhile, combine all the tahini sauce ingredients in
a bowl with 1 tablespoon of water – you may need more
if the mixture thickens (you want a yoghurt-like
consistency).

Serve the cauliflower florets with the tahini sauce
drizzled over and scattered with the pomegranate seeds
and fresh herbs.

DIPS

I am all about quick and nutritious ideas, and dips make a
great healthy snack, always ready to go. They're also
great to add to family-style sharing plates if people are
coming over.

These dips take minutes to make, are high in protein
and fibre and taste great with a selection of crudités. You
can leave out the garlic with any of these recipes if it's
not your thing.

HUMMUS

1 x 400g tin chickpeas, rinsed and drained
2 garlic cloves
3 tbsp tahini
1 tbsp olive oil
Juice of 1 lemon
Pinch of paprika
Sea salt

Whizz the chickpeas, garlic, tahini, olive oil and lemon juice together in a blender to the consistency you prefer. Add some salt to taste and serve garnished with a sprinkling of paprika.

BUTTERBEAN DIP

This is the same recipe as the hummus, above, using butterbeans (or any tinned beans) in place of the chickpeas.

AVOCADO DIP

Everyone loves a guacamole. Follow the instructions for the avocado in the Mexican Salad recipe on page 223. You can add herbs and/or red onions or finely chopped tomatoes.

And don't forget a squeeze of fresh lime juice and lime zest, too.

COCKTAILS

Tequila ... it makes me happy. We've all heard the song, right? (Well, if it doesn't, it certainly should!) But if, like me, you spend a lot of time and energy trying to get in shape for summer, you'll probably not be thrilled about all the calories lurking in our favourite summer drinks.

I'm not suggesting for a minute that we all go teetotal – no no, God forbid! – it's just about making clever choices. This is where tequila comes in.

When it comes to alcohol-induced bloating, tequila helps to control the absorption of fat, so won't leave you feeling sluggish like your favourite beer or wine. Being a cleaner alcohol, tequila means you can wave goodbye to your hangovers, too – trust me, I've tried it and it works!

When I first started seeing my facial acupuncturist, Sarah, she advised me that if I was to drink I should choose tequila due to its lower sugar content, which makes it better for the skin (that's when I knew she and I would be friends for life!) – such good advice.

So, it's important to choose your tipple wisely and always drink in moderation. And as I mentioned earlier in the book, if alcohol doesn't agree with you any more, be honest with yourself and just cut it out of your life.

THE MINIMAL MARGARITA

This is the simplest way to mix your tequila. Use a natural sweetener, such as honey or agave syrup (I like to use this, and it has even less sugar than honey), then squeeze in a fresh lime, lots of ice, shake it up and voila!

My new fave variation is a watermelon margarita. Simply blend fresh watermelon (remove the pips first), then add tequila blanco and a little agave to sweeten if you like – although I find it's usually sweet enough without. It's honestly so delicious, wonderfully refreshing and cools down the skin. The only downside is that it's so easy to drink. You have been warned!

TEQUILA AND SODA

The least calorific way to enjoy tequila – simply mix with fizzy or soda water and a lime wedge. What better way to stay hydrated (in moderation)!

SKINNY PALOMA

The paloma is Mexico's favourite drink. This grapefruit-juice-based cocktail is packed full of vitamin C, which helps to maintain a healthy heart – just what the doctor ordered! Simply mix fresh grapefruit juice with sparkling water, a twist of lime and your chosen tequila.

BLOODY MARIA

The day after the night before, if you're partial to a Bloody Mary at brunch or even breakfast (no judgement), swap out the vodka for a tequila blanco and it's a Bloody Maria!

So, there you have it, my guide to enjoying a calorie-friendly tipple. My advice would be to get a decent-quality tequila – and remember to always drink responsibly.

But if the tequila doesn't work and your libido is lost and can't be found, read on …

SEX

Or lack of.

If this subject makes you extremely uncomfortable, or you find yourself cringing or squirming at its mention, skip this section and come back to it when you are ready to revisit. There's absolutely no judgement – I promise, none – as some people just don't want to talk about it or disclose or discuss anything about their own sexual experiences or sex lives in general, let alone hear about someone else's.

If you are a family member of mine, maybe this chapter is also not for you, as I will be going on a deep dive (pun intended) into my experiences with sex over the years and how it has shaped and formed a lot of the opinions I have about myself. But for those of you who want to stick it out with me here, I hope it will offer some lightness surrounding this topic, as well as some help and advice on getting our confidence and, in turn, the jiggy-jiggy back on track, if that tempts you at all.

For so many years sex, for me, was about validation. I have always been slightly underwhelmed by the activity itself, though, if I am honest; I feel like it's something we all have such high expectations about, then, when it happens, it's like, seriously – what's all the fuss about? I never really experienced much satisfaction in my late teens or my twenties; if the person I was with was enjoying it, that for me was enough, which I obviously now know is not what it's all about. For an awfully long time, I was a people pleaser; I think that's a role that we women easily fall into.

It is so sad to have realised this only recently, in the last ten or so years – or maybe I have always known but been too scared to admit it or do something about changing it.

I can look back and say that I most definitely had sex when I didn't really want it and I felt pressured into it. I have also had some ugly experiences with men, and on reflection, I do feel that I was taken advantage of in a way that I should have been more aware of and been more attuned to. This book is not about that, although I do hope to confront the people concerned one day and tell them how they made me feel. It is frustrating, as I should have known better and had more conviction about what I wanted or, more importantly, did not want.

Now, don't be mistaken, I wasn't sleeping around with any Tom, Dick or Harry. I found myself in many long-term relationships. However, sadly, these were mostly with narcissistic, insecure, arrogant men who certainly loved themselves more than they could ever have loved me. I never felt that they cared for me at all. The sex itself was average at best, very wham-bam-thank-you-ma'am, with little consideration of what I may have wanted and most certainly no tenderness or that key ingredient: love. I was there simply to accommodate their desires and that was pretty much it. They could have been bashing a hole in the wall as far as I was concerned.

I didn't know any different, though. You don't when you are younger, do you? Especially if your first few years of having sex are without compassion or care either from the person you're sleeping with or from yourself. I realise as I write this that things could have been different. I had someone who I thought was a lovely first boyfriend, who seemed normal. That is, until he cheated on me and broke my heart (a pattern that played out with a few other boyfriends, too).

In the beginning, it was all very innocent; we didn't sleep together as such, both being virgins and too afraid, but he used to lie on top of me, both of us fully dressed, kissing and dry humping. This used to feel amazing, and I used to orgasm every time. We both did. It was very pure, very innocent and we were both very into each other. (I have since discussed this with quite a few women and we agree that we should bring back the dry humping, as it is never not satisfying. To this day, I still can't climax through penetrative sex alone; like everything, sex is very subjective.) These were some of the most exciting and passionate times, when both of us felt connected and focused on our bodies grinding together, not a worry in the world. It felt incredible.

So, imagine my disappointment when I did eventually lose my virginity in the most unromantic, unloving way. It was not with my first boyfriend, but with the school stud (or at least he thought he was). I was desperate for the cool boy in school to like me, and so desperate to no longer be a virgin at sixteen, and sadly that set the precedent for the rest of my life. That need for validation ...

I used sex to feel connected, to feel loved, needed and appreciated, and it was always the men who seemed to enjoy it much more than I did. There were times when the biggest thrill for me was the sense of control, of being desired, of being wanted – that was the turn-on. But being deeply insecure with no self-worth is a dangerous and destructive combination, one that is a red flag to a narcissistic bull. They can sniff it a mile away.

It has taken me so many years to figure all this out. To find my sense of self-worth, to figure out what I deserve and what I want from a partner, not just in the bedroom but in life. Therefore, writing this book feels important because I would like to prevent anyone else from coming to this realisation so late (or too late) in life. It has shaped who I am now, what I stand for and what my boundaries are, but it has taken a very long time.

I think what I have written so far implies that I didn't enjoy sex at all – far from it, though. I really enjoyed it. I was never into one-night stands (or at least, not too many of them) but I certainly enjoyed myself. I love the physicality of it, the contact and the animal attraction. I was, of course, deeply attracted to the opposite sex, and sometimes to the same sex, and I would be lying if I said I hadn't experimented a little; that was fun, and I certainly have no regrets.

A friend the other day told me that a lot of women who are now in the menopause or are slightly older and who are attracted to women are acting on it, as they feel they no longer need men. And I kind of understand it. They perhaps no longer have that primal need to procreate and start a family, and sleeping with women can be a much more sensual, more gentle, more intense and more giving experience. There is an understanding about what feels good and what our needs are.

For those in healthy, happy heterosexual relationships, or even gay or bisexual ones, being perimenopausal and menopausal can throw a big spanner in the works when it comes to sex in general. The first thing I can pick out – and what was certainly key for me – is the lack of confidence due to body changes. As I have already said, my weight gain and the sheer daily exhaustion didn't exactly make me feel like the sexiest person in the world. I know that when I get into bed these days, the last thing I feel like doing is having sex – for a number of reasons, but mainly because my libido just isn't what it used to be. When I am knackered, spooning and snuggling are pure bliss for me and can be just as good. I tend to fall asleep as soon as possible, curled up together. That, for me, is a good night in.

Also, through my perimenopausal years, each time I had sex, I would usually end up with a bladder infection. It was so utterly painful and I could not help but feel beyond angry and frustrated. I would then, of course, have to go to the doctor or late-night pharmacy to get medication to help me heal. It stopped being fun and definitely didn't seem worth it. I always knew the outcome – it would be the same story, and I would end up in pain, quite depressed and low about it. It stopped me from feeling any desire for penetrative sex. I would prefer to fool around without the act of actual sex, as I was terrified it would leave me peeing blood again. You understand why, right?

If you're in a new relationship or trying out something new, as long as it makes you truly happy and gives you satisfaction, I think good on you. I am all for a healthy, happy, rampant sex life, and in a relationship, I do think it's important, as connection and intimacy are crucial. And for many of us women, it goes deeper than attraction or a physical thing – I would say it's mainly a mental thing. Men don't seem to have to connect on both levels – although this, I know, is not a revelation.

What I have learned is that it's to do with the old hormones again or, in the case of those of us going into perimenopause or menopause, the lack of them. When our oestrogen levels start to dip, as well as our testosterone, it affects every part of our bodies, our minds and our vaginas.

Everyone's perimenopause and menopause journeys are unique. I suffered with extreme anxiety, depression and weight gain that left me feeling less attractive, far less confident about my body and much less sexual. In addition, I didn't know it at the time, but my testosterone levels were depleted, leaving me exhausted, with no energy whatsoever and no desire for sex. I would urge you to get these hormone levels checked and tested to see what you need to do next to redress the balance, particularly if you are feeling any of these symptoms.

I was also majorly sleep deprived, as my body temperature ranged from extreme inferno heat to shivering cold, swinging back and forth between the two all through the night. Let's just say it wasn't the ideal mood setter for a long night of passion, especially if I was up every hour having to pee. At my very worst, I wasn't getting much sleep at all, and I felt like a shadow of my former self. I was short-tempered and would fly into a rage at the drop of a hat. My poor George. Even if I would have been up for a roll around between the sheets, I don't think he would have wanted to come near me. I was like a woman possessed.

The lack of oestrogen also means that we experience changes in our vaginas and vulvas. Where once they were juicy, plump and accommodating, the vaginal walls thick and rich with blood vessels, they now become more sensitive, much drier, the skin thinner and prone to tearing and ripping. This can cause uncomfortable, painful sex, usually for me (and many other women) resulting in a bladder infection, as mentioned above. Plus, I remember before I got on to the correct HRT, I lost all sensitivity around my clitoris – so even if I'd wanted to have an orgasm, it was near impossible (or if I did manage, it was not satisfying at all). Not the best advertisement for a session, is it?

Apologies if I am making you squirm; it's not my intention. But I just want to address this subject as honestly as I can because there is so much pressure on us girls as we get older. I have heard from many friends who talk about the crazy, wild sex they are having, swinging from the chandeliers, having earth-shattering orgasms every night, and as much as I am happy for them, it does make me feel inadequate. The pressure we put on ourselves intensifies, as well as obviously wanting to keep the people in our lives happy by performing between the sheets.

There is light at the end of the tunnel, though, I promise. There is help for us all, and once you get that help and take the pressure off somewhat, sex will become more attractive again, and you will feel like a sexual being once more. My advice is that it must be more on your terms – with lower lighting and a more patient, tender lover. B' wait, there is more ...

So, what else can we do to get our groove back? Firstly, oestrogen. This is going to help with any vaginal dryness and soreness – these issues fall under the term vaginal atrophy, and some women even find wearing jeans or riding a bike completely unbearable. You'll find lots more information about this on page 259.

There are also some amazing toys to help stimulate and get you more in the mood, awakening that part of you that you had maybe forgotten existed, and getting the juices and the inspiration flowing. They are inconspicuous and don't look like medieval torture devices – all fantastic additions in the bedroom, not intimidating and nothing that looks like a huge rabbit with bells, lights and whistles (the last thing I would want). These gentle clitoral stimulators have made sex enjoyable again, doing wonders for turning up the fizz. I was introduced to the Womaniser, a rather discreet and elegant-looking clitoral stimulator that has truly changed my life. It kind of blows and sucks and feels so bloody good, I am not going to lie; I really like it. My advice is to look online, there are so many great websites offering so many different versions that you will find something you fancy. Just be brave, dive in and experiment with

tion is key in any loving and long-term rela-
able to explain to our partners what
what is lacking, say how we are feel-
rtantly, be confident to ask for what we

want. Sometimes it's about going back to basics to work out what does turn us on. Maybe watching some porn together, experimenting with new toys, having a drink to help relax. I find wearing sexy underwear helps to get me in the mood, as well as making me feel more sexual, more confident and equally turned on. It all has to start with honesty, and I know that can be so tricky to bring up. Maybe over a candlelit dinner and a glass of wine, or after a night out together, throw caution to the wind and show your partner something you have been reading that has turned you on, or a film or a scene that had given you a little twinge, a fire between your legs or has got the juices flowing.

There is some great underwear out there, whatever your body shape and in all sizes, that can complement and flatter areas we may have concerns about as we get older. You can order it online to be delivered to your home address, try it on comfortably without any pressure, with nice mirrors and lighting instead of a cold changing room.

If you need some courage to reconnect with the sensual part of yourself, or even just to look at your body, believe me, you wouldn't be the first. I know that feeling; you are not alone. But remember to appreciate your body for what it is, however it has changed over the years, and practise the self-acceptance we discussed earlier in the book (see page 116).

If you're uncomfortable or unhappy about your tummy area, I highly recommend basques, lacy bodies and shapewear. To lift sagging breasts, you can use brilliantly designed push-up balconette bras in assorted styles (keep them on for the whole night, if that makes you feel sexier – I do!). And hold-ups or suspenders make legs look longer and slimmer. A small but important reminder is to make sure you get the right size, so they fit you well and aren't too small, as that is a total confidence crusher. I know this all too well from my own experience of trying to dress up using underwear I bought a hundred years ago. The end result was that I didn't look great and didn't even dare to come out of the bedroom – the opposite of the intended effect. Personally, I would always opt for underwear that you love and feel good in, rather than trying to please your partner with what you think they might like. Even better, you could go shopping together, which is a fun and sexy thing to do. I really enjoy the anticipation of us making time for each other and preparing for a cheeky night in, adding a spark of excitement – all so simple, yet so important in a relationship.

All these things can be brilliant at breaking the ice and spicing up your sex life. It's important to be brave and remember how it used to be before kids, marriage and menopause. When you had fewer inhibitions and just went for it. A little bit of this must come back out to play, especially if you want to reignite the va va voom in the bedroom.

But maybe the bedroom is the problem? Perhaps being more inventive with locations is the key to getting back into that groove. If you have, perhaps, always wanted to have sex in a car or somewhere risky, bring that up – talk about it. You'd be surprised how even just raising it as a suggestion can sometimes be enough to get you both fired up, even if you never act upon it. (But if you do, please be careful not to get arrested – and if that does happen, do not blame me.) All joking aside, sex in places outside of the bedroom can be extremely fun and exciting. So, say yes to discussing fantasies. Sex is about mental stimulation as well as physical, so just say it and try not to recoil in shame.

If you have ever had any fantasies that involve S&M, being a dominatrix, any kinky curiosities, I truly believe you should explore and bring them to the table. I think your partner might wholeheartedly embrace it. If you have always loved the thought of being tied up, or tying your partner up, buy some silk ropes or scarves to use on one another. If you like the thought of your eyes being covered – the mystery of the unknown of what they might do to you – throw that into the mix. Basically, experiment and have some fun. Role play can be fun, dressing up can be fun, sex should be fun. So, don't forget the humour of it all, the funny side; if one of you suggests something new or you decide to try a new position and if in the middle of it all, it just seems ridiculous, laugh it off. Remember, as long as it is consensual and no one gets hurt, go for it.

Soft lighting adds to the atmosphere and helps me to feel so much more confident. I don't have any spotlights anywhere, as this is by far the most unflattering light and no one, I repeat no one, looks good standing or lying under a spotlight. Candle and soft bulbs in lamps are good, but for me it's just candlelight, which is sensual, erotic and, most importantly, flattering.

Music always creates a pleasant atmosphere, or if you're feeling brave, then I'd suggest a naughty movie or some porn – you have free licence here to choose what makes you tick and turns you on. It's good sometimes to show each other what you like and to start to play with either yourself or each other. And remember the good lube!

If the thought of playing with yourself fills you with total horror, let's delve deeper. I think most of us discover self-love or masturbation in our teens. Families and cultures can impact the shame that surrounds it and that can stay with us, making us feel as if we are doing something wrong, something dirty. But it is totally natural and no one should be ashamed of it. This is, after all, the way you first discover how you like to be touched and what works for you. It can also really enhance your sex life by showing your partner what you like. And, of course, it helps to get the juices flowing and the vagina throbbing and excited for more.

One thing I know is that if you don't use it, you lose it, meaning that if you don't make the effort, it will all just go out of the window and you will never be bothered to get that energy or that spark between the sheets back again. Maybe, like me, you're just too tired all the time, but even if you have to schedule in time for sex, so be it. Otherwise, you will just become good friends and that can cause you either to drift apart, losing that intimacy and connection, and/or start to look elsewhere, neither of which you want to happen. So, dig deep and make the effort.

THE BENEFITS OF THE BIG O

Let's talk orgasms. Not all orgasms are the same, as there are different ways to climax, and everyone is unique. Clitoral climax is the most common and, as the name suggests, it requires stimulation of the clitoris, where there is a bundle of nerve endings, and where sensitivity and arousal are experienced when it is touched, rubbed, kissed and played with. Vaginal orgasms, as you may have guessed, occur by stimulation inside the vagina. Not every woman can achieve this kind, except maybe by using certain toys, or G-spot stimulators.

I will reiterate that being pre- and post-menopause can have a huge impact on body image, body confidence and affect the quality of orgasms or the ability to orgasm at all, but please persevere; orgasms are so good for you and a necessary part of your wellbeing. The vaginal contractions that occur deep inside when you climax are fantastic at helping with pelvic-floor health. I see it as the ultimate act of self-care, and whether you stimulate the clitoris or however you like to climax, the most important thing is that you do have an orgasm. Incorporating self-pleasure, masturbation – whatever you want to call it – is my twice-weekly prescription for you (or daily, if you prefer). It truly is so important for your mental and physical wellbeing and there are so many other health benefits, too.

When you orgasm, a flood of chemicals, as well as the hormones oestrogen and testosterone, are released into your brain. These help with a whole host of issues: oestrogen aids the building blocks of skin, helping to produce more collagen and blood flow to the scalp, which, in turn, encourages hair to grow and skin to glow. Testosterone can really help with mental and emotional wellbeing, and the chemicals dopamine and oxytocin improve mood and lower stress, reducing cortisol production (cortisol is a stress trigger and causes inflammation within the body). As an added bonus, sleep is also improved. These chemicals help with pain, too, as well as lowering levels of anxiety, improving cognitive function and boosting immunity. Basically, what's not to love about orgasms?

I really hope that even if you and your partner are not having sex at this moment in time, you are at least pleasuring yourself. I've said it before and I'll say it again – my prescription for you is to try to climax at least once a week to keep everything happy and healthy in your body.

As much as I know I need to practise what I preach, I have to be honest that these days, getting into bed and just snuggling with George is one of my favourite things in the world to do, as I mentioned earlier. I love the intimacy of being close together, our bodies huddled up, holding hands or feet entwined and feeling exhausted yet content after a productive day. I also realise that the stresses of life and making money take it all out of us and leave us somewhat preoccupied, so that some nights, by the time we fall into bed, I am asleep as soon as my head hits the pillow – and as someone who struggled with sleep throughout the peri-menopause years, I have to weigh up what I prefer!

For me, holidays are good for reconnecting, away from the pressure of the alarm clock going off. But I will go back to what I said previously – communication is key and if you're both communicating, and you talk to each other about what you need, what you want, what you feel you're missing and what you really desire, that's where the real intimacy lies.

SEX AND DESIRE

BY DR CHARLOTTE GOODING, GP AND MENOPAUSE SPECIALIST

Midlife can be a time of change for our sexuality, i.e., the way we think, feel and behave around sex. In the same way that physical changes can impact our sexual function, so can changes in our minds. So, it's just as important that we address these, as well as the physical issues, to improve intimacy and sex in midlife.

Things I want you to know:

It's OK for desire not to be spontaneous

There are different types of desire: responsive desire, which is often triggered by touch, closeness and sexual contact, and spontaneous desire – the one often portrayed to us in films, books, even art, where there is a spontaneous eruption or spark for sex that comes out of the blue. It's important to align ourselves with the reality that desire is not always spontaneous and can fluctuate, particularly in long-term relationships. Our worries about not feeling spontaneous desire can often lead to discomfort around sex in a relationship, and sex can become the elephant in the room, leading us to avoid physical affection in all its forms with our partners in case it leads to sex. However, small, intimate behaviours such as handholding and kissing can help us to trigger the other type of desire –

responsive desire – when we accept there is no pressure for it to lead somewhere.

Remove the pressure

Pressure to have sex and to be intimate can put a huge brake on desire by shutting down our openness to connect. Responsive desire needs time to set up and for us to feel connected. This can be through the way we interact and how open we are to connection with our partners, and by exploring the reasons why we want to be intimate – is it to connect, or feel attractive or loved? Knowing that we don't always need to have sex to fulfil those needs can remove the pressure to do so.

Less can be more!

The frequency of sex is not important, but the quality of it is – it's better to have sex less often but for it to give pleasure than to have it all the time and be unsatisfying, especially as we know that sex gives a pleasure reward and is what relation-ships need to thrive.

Focus on pleasure

Particularly for females, pleasure is not taught and is often surrounded by taboo. Find what gives you pleasure – experi-ment with various levels of touch, temperature, etc., but also look more broadly at what brings you pleasure in life – it might just be a cup of tea in bed! If you can open yourself up to experiencing pleasure in general, without any pressure or guilt attached, you will be more open to it in the bedroom.

Go off script

Many of us follow an ingrained script of what sex should look like from what we see, read or from our previous sexual experiences. Try going with the flow, be guided by what feels good and explore without judgement and open up your experiences by reading or listening to different narratives about sex.

Talk about it

The taboo around sex means we often don't talk about it with our partners. If you are worried about talking to your partner about sex, ask yourself why and start to explore where that fear is coming from.

Be in the moment

We live such busy lives, and we adopt so many different roles that we are often distracted from our own feelings and emotions. It can be hard to give ourselves fully to intimate experiences as we run through the mental to-do lists or just the many thoughts that take up our head space. A regular five–ten-minute daily mindfulness practice can help us to learn to get out of our heads and focus on the sensations of sex and our desires.

Oestrogen

Declining oestrogen levels in the perimenopause and meno-pause can have a huge impact on the vulval and vaginal tissues, as well as the pelvic floor, the bladder and the urethra. We call this genito-urinary syndrome of the menopause (GSM). All women will experience these changes to some degree, but only very few seek help for troublesome symptoms.

Low oestrogen causes a change in the vaginal pH, which become less acidic and can disrupt the vaginal microbiome, and the vaginal and vulval tissues can become thin and dry. Many women have discomfort in the vulva and some find it so debilitating they cannot wear underwear, sit down comfortably or enjoy things like riding a bike, as the vulval tissues become thin and fragile. This can also affect sex, and lots of women find sex painful, often describing a burning or stinging sensation inside the vagina and particularly around the entrance to the vaginal canal where the skin is very thin. The friction of sex can cause micro tears and some women may experience bleeding (any bleeding during or after sex must be reported to your doctor). The bladder and urethra can also be affected by low oestrogen and women can experience symptoms of leaking urine or increasingly needing to pass urine, as well as increased urinary-tract infections.

Treatment of GSM starts with good vulval care. There is no need to wash the vagina – it is self-cleaning and vaginal douching/steaming can cause disruption to the sensitive vaginal microbiome, leading to more issues. Treat the vulva like you would your favourite cashmere sweater – with great care! Wash delicately and at low heat, avoid harsh chemicals and dry gently.

For sex, a good lubricant is a must! I recommend YES lubricants, which can come as oil-based or water-based. A good tip to reduce discomfort during sex can be to use a technique called double glide, where one partner uses a water-based lubricant and the other an oil-based one; as oil and water don't mix, this reduces friction and makes for more comfortable sex – it can be a real game changer! (Remember, though, that oil-based lubricants must not be used with condoms as they can damage the Latex.)

Vaginal moisturisers can also be used. These differ from lubricants as they are longer lasting and designed to replace moisture in the vulval and vaginal tissues. These can be used as frequently as needed. Ingredients really matter here, so avoid any that may cause irritation (you don't need any more of that!), such as glycerine, glycol, perfumes, parabens and alcohol. Oestrogen can be replaced in the vulval and vaginal tissues using local topical oestrogens in the form of pessaries, gels, creams and even a ring. These can be prescribed by your doctor or nurse, and one type of vaginal oestrogen pessary, GINA, can be bought over the counter.

Issues with pain during sex can affect our ability to enjoy it and have a huge impact on libido or any desire to have sex or any intimacy in the first place. It's therefore so important to seek help if you are experiencing pain, as it can have a much wider impact on your sex life.

ADVICE FOR LOVED ONES

Something that I feel is missing when it comes to the menopause is guidance and advice for our loved ones.

This is a hard enough time for us women to go through, let alone be able to communicate how we feel to the people around us; we feel lost and alone, so it makes sense that we leave our loved ones in the dark about this time.

It's heartbreaking that a lot of families go through a turbulent, testing time – teenagers arguing with their mums, partners feeling completely at their wits' end, not understanding how to talk to their loved ones or how to approach them, seeing the person they love and have lived with for years change before their eyes.

Another area that causes heartache is living with guilt because of the confusing things happening to us, the uncontrollable, angry, emotional eruptions, those times when we just want to lock ourselves away from the people we love. This perpetuates the cycle of anxiety and even more guilt, eating away at us – and it's all so unnecessary.

As I mentioned before, we really do need education about this subject in schools; we need to accept that this is an inevitable stage in a woman's life – something that directly affects 51 per cent of the global population, and indirectly affects partners, colleagues and family members, too.

So, this isn't just a woman's problem – it is a societal issue, and the sooner we are all up to speed in recognising signs and symptoms, the happier the world will be. We all need to appreciate that there might be a few wobbles for a woman in her forties, fifties and sixties that they can't always put their fingers on and understand that having insight and empathy and trying to be gentler, more supportive and more sensitive is going to really help everybody.

The emotional anguish on all parts is devastating, so I wanted to tackle this subject with delicacy, by speaking to the person who has handled my menopause in the most positive and supportive way: my rock, George.

I was curious to know what was going on in *his* head when the angry, emotional outbursts happened, usually out of the blue, when I would literally attack him verbally, sometimes spitefully. I wanted to know from somebody who has never had to live through this kind of experience before or even understand this time in a woman's life, how he managed to navigate it and realise that there was something going on that wasn't just me having some kind of breakdown.

So, let's talk to George.

LISA: George, can I ask you to cast your mind back to eight or nine years ago – what you thought was happening to me when, say, we got home from a lovely dinner, having had a lovely time, and then just as we were getting home, I would switch and turn into a completely different person, screaming and shouting. What did you think was happening to me?

GEORGE: It's a great question. I think the most important thing is I guess I've sort of been taught in life, for as long as I can remember from my parents, that spontaneous actions aren't necessarily a fair indication of somebody's character, and when this whole journey began, while, of course, it was a little shocking, it wasn't ever impossible to sort out or to start to rationalise that things were becoming more difficult for you. To work through it was a simple decision for me; it was about making a positive commitment to be there for you.

LISA: So you just knew instinctively that it was hormonal? Or did you think that it was maybe me being overworked, overstretched, and it was a stress reaction? Did you ever consider at any time, I can't handle this woman – she is irrational and angry, and I don't like it and I can't seem to make her happy?

GEORGE: I never felt any of those things. I
knew that it wasn't you and I knew that because
I believed in our relationship, I had to be
there to support you through whatever was
going on.

The worst sort of support is to interrogate.
What you were going through required love and a
sense of safety, and I wanted to make sure those
were there in the relationship.

My advice to anybody who is in a similar
situation to me would be this: don't judge the
person on the moment; instead, think about the
broader picture. It's my belief that you live life
going forwards (as in, you are not conscious of
necessarily understanding things as they happen),
but you understand life backwards. In other
words, you reflect on the past, so if you try to
make a judgement or try to understand what's
happening now, then you're probably going to
end up with a flawed reality, judged on somebody
else's actions that you know not to be true. I
didn't ever want to judge you on what you were
dealing with, and I never have.

LISA: What would you say to people who are living
with somebody who is changing before their eyes
and they feel unable to get through to them, to
even just talk to them?

Maybe this person has been misdiagnosed for years, maybe they've been diagnosed with depression, and it's got to the point where they just can't communicate with one another any more. Maybe the person who's dealing with menopausal symptoms doesn't know what's happening and has shut everybody else out – their kids, their partner, everyone.

What advice would you give in this situation, because it is a lonely place for both parties?

GEORGE: I think if you're in a relationship and you know it's the right one, then you know that person – and in knowing that person, you understand what's them, and what isn't them. I think first and foremost that any partner of somebody who is on that peri- or menopausal journey must judge it from their point of view. You need to be present, make a safe environment, don't make them feel like they're going crazy, avoid the sorts of triggers and anxiety that are already going for them – they don't need to be in a place of judgement or a place of critique; they don't need any of those places that make them reflect on themselves in a bad way.

Again, you need to provide a safe space that is to the benefit of everybody in the relationship.

And the second thing is, yes, you must start to understand what is going on.

I'll be honest, you were the one who highlighted what was happening to you because you've been so interested in both understanding the changes you were experiencing from your point of view and realising that there was a role for you, given your profile – that you could disseminate and communicate the relevant information in a way that made sense to other women. Others who were also on this difficult-to-navigate path going forwards.

So, again, I would recommend creating a safe place with no judgement and realise you have to communicate together and talk about it – not in terms of the bad things that happen but the progress that is being made about how you are understanding things better. And anybody who thinks that this is just one conversation is crazy. It takes a long time, but in the context of the overall time of your relationship, this is just a very small interlude, and getting on that journey together builds a stronger bond between you.

LISA: Thank you. I know we are very lucky because you do have so much patience and understanding, so we have been able to communicate, to talk things through – plus, as you said, I had to go out and investigate what was happening to me, even though it took a good six years to really nail down the right prescription and help I needed professionally.

We never got to the point that I know so many couples reach, where they just want to give up. I hear from people who are at breaking point and it upsets me so much, as when you are living through it, it feels like hell on earth – for everyone, I suspect.

I know what it feels like to want to push people away, to feel hate and irritation and be violent verbally like I was to you, the person I love; the irrational behaviour that is honestly uncontrollable.

GEORGE: My advice is always going to be based on my own understanding and time is the key for me. You must look at time not in minutes and hours, but how you deal with each of those moments, and look at the bigger picture – have that aerial view, that awareness of the fact that this is not going to be for ever.

Support, don't judge. Create that safe space and know you can't ask the question 'How long will this last?' or expect there to be a moment when it suddenly stops. If you can't get your head around that, you need to think harder about what time means to you.

I know we partners in the relationship are not having to deal with it; it's not as hard for us and we need to take a very positive, supportive role. We can stand alongside and keep a relationship moving in the same sort of direction, and it will be a stronger, more resilient relationship. We, the partners, need to think about the bigger picture, have more awareness of our expectations. The partner's role is to offer support, non-judgement, security.

I think the other point is to focus on the good things, the good times – enjoying meals out, going for walks, mini breaks, whatever it is – just grabbing twenty minutes and going for a coffee, cooking together or having a dance together to your favourite music (or something that, you know, maybe you don't like but the other person does). Whatever it is, live for the moment and have fun celebrating those things.

Be confident that the relationship is going to get stronger.

LISA: Thank you so much, my love. I obviously feel very blessed that you have this incredible attitude and that you've been able to see it not as a direct attack on you. I'm so grateful that you always saw the bigger picture.

Now we're kind of through it and out the other

end (even though you don't go through the menopause, you go into it), we have gained a whole new lease of life, and you can vouch for women once they have got ownership on what's happening to them, once they understand the changes.

Hopefully, by reading this book, by recognising things that maybe make them stressed and anxious, by removing related toxicity and triggers from their lives, others can see that the best is yet to come. That this is most definitely the beginning and not the end of their lives or relationships.

GEORGE: Yeah, I totally agree. The future is so bright, and I think we're all just getting started. And, yeah, I think if you approach every day with that mentality, regardless of how old you are, it's a hell of a powerful thing. That contribution to society, those relationships with others and – most importantly – with yourself are in your gift, and they are free. It is all about mindset, and it makes a difference to what happens tomorrow. So have faith and be kind to each other.

We've Got This

We are just getting started!

I am just getting started, that I know for sure. It feels so liberating to honestly believe this in my very being. I am at the beginning of an exciting new chapter in life, a brand new road that I am going down with all the knowledge from my years so far to guide me and protect me.

We all evolve and we are constantly growing. The intelligence and awareness I personally have gained over the last fifty years – the bruises, the scars as well – help me to move forwards with conviction and carve out a beautiful future, one that I can visualise, one that I have manifested and one that I deserve.

I am taking forwards with me a fountain of knowledge, saying goodbye to things and situations that no longer serve me, stepping away from bad or unhealthy habits and living in the here and now. I am moving away from drama, from people or situations that have caused me to feel either unhappy or ill at ease. I am embarking on new adventures, which involve exploration, finding new places, better communication and more connections. I am continuing to heal through daily rituals, weekly routines, knowing what I need to do to feed my body, mind and soul.

After reading this book, I hope that you will be loving who you are, and who you have become. Be proud of how far you have come and what you have achieved and take time to acknowledge the tiny wins (or huge ones) when you look around at your life.

There will always be people who, on the surface, seem to have more than we do – mainly material things, like a bigger house or a sporty car – and while they might appear to be less stressed, that's rarely the case, as more money doesn't necessarily equal zero stress, and sometimes it causes a lot more.

Our inner happiness is worth all the gold and riches in the world. We should value our minds and freedom of movement for our bodies and, most importantly, surround ourselves with love and nourish ourselves with health and happiness and the people we love. And if they are no longer with us here on earth, we must treasure the beautiful, long-lasting memories of precious times together, and highlight the importance of those deep connections. And love the people around us even harder.

I have purged the hurt and pain that I squashed deep down inside over the years, repressing it for so long and hiding it away from everyone – even from myself – as I rolled with the ebbs and flows of life. I embrace the changes within, and those on the surface, too – the softness around my eyes, the lines of a life lived, like the changing of the seasons. I no longer need validation from others, only from myself.

I am moving forward with a new future – less party, more purpose. The positives of becoming older and entering a second spring are enormous, and I am taking ownership of the worldly wisdom I have gathered and the acceptance I now have.

However old you are reading this, think back to how quickly the years have passed. Life is short, and it's a gift, so let's sprinkle some magic over our days and really appreciate it. It's time to park that negative shit, shrug off the crap, the damaging comparisons and insecurities and put it all to bed. Wave farewell and good riddance to all that!

A SUMMARY OF MY MIDLIFE MUSINGS

Here's some of what I've learned over the years.

ROUTINE

Babies need it, children thrive on it and I know that I am happier and calmer when I have it in my life. At first, I thought this meant that I was boring (or that life was), but routine is good, it is necessary and it works. Our brains respond so well to it – the simplicity of having a plan and sticking with it. When I get out of routine, that is when things have the capacity to spiral.

Waking up at roughly the same time each day, drinking hot water with lemon, doing a workout, taking a daily walk to your regular coffee spot, having breakfast, doing yoga or breathwork – whatever you do, keep up that routine and you will thank yourself for it.

DO WHAT YOU WANT TO DO

I have said it before and I will say it again: listen to your intuition.

It sounds selfish and self-centred, but as we get older, we really must be truer to ourselves. If you don't want to do something, go somewhere or see someone, then don't. Simple.

SLEEP

We need it. Good sleep hygiene is imperative, which means having a good wind-down routine, a cool, uncluttered place to sleep, keeping the lighting low, the sheets breathable, and pillow sprays and oils at the ready.

I like to also take magnesium before bed, to help my muscles and my mind unwind and switch off. Try not to drink too much or too late in the day, otherwise you might be up all night peeing.

WRITE LISTS

This is the easiest way to keep up with what is happening day to day, week by week, to keep a handle on things as they change, and what you must do.

Do not beat yourself up if you don't always get to the end of the list with everything ticked off. Just start a new list for the next day and simply add those to-dos to it.

If your mind is racing, get that shit down on paper, whatever is in your head. Get a nice notebook to keep beside your bed – it's a great tool for offloading on those early mornings or late nights when your head is whirling. Scribble down your worries, dreams, desires, ambitions or things to do and then it's out of your head and on the paper. This brings me lots of calm, and that feeling of being organised is blissful.

BE KIND TO YOURSELF

How often do you say unkind things to yourself? Things you would never say to your friends or loved ones. So, why be so hurtful to yourself? Instead, thank your body for what it does for you daily, continually and mostly without appreciation, and get into the habit of treating yourself to a daily dose of thanks and gratitude.

HAVE A DUVET DAY

Sometimes you've just got to chill, no pressure. It's important to listen to what your body is telling you and take time to recharge. Enjoy those days, switch off, stay off your phone and devices, and give your brain a total go-slow. Relax.

TAKE A SOCIAL MEDIA HOLIDAY

Take a break or maybe delete the apps or accounts. You can always reactivate them!

THE POWER OF SAYING NO

The power you will feel saying no to anything that does not serve you – the incredible feeling that will envelop you when you stay true to what you want or need – is beyond liberating. It took me a long time to do this, so my advice is to start now.

FIND NEW WAYS TO HAVE FUN

Are there any hobbies or interests that have you always wanted to do or learn? Well, start now – take control. Yes, that first class or introduction might feel a little scary or intimidating, but after that initial step, you'll be so proud of pushing yourself. How about joining a book club, or starting dance lessons, art classes or a reflexology course? I would like to study for a qualification in nutrition, as well as learn a language – but whatever it is that you have always wanted to do, do it. You are never too old to learn something new. More strings to your bow, I say!

DECLUTTER

We all need to do it. Having a good old sort out does wonders for your mental health. It makes more space in your life, plus, having a good clear out and giving to others is extremely rewarding.

Make three piles: one for things to keep, one to give to friends or family and one for charity. Giving away things that you forgot you had because they were tucked away in a drawer or at the back of a cupboard could really make someone else's day. So let them enjoy that dress you have worn so many times before or that clutch bag that no longer suits your style. Tidying up is so therapeutic, as you feel lighter and more organised. Plus, you can then see what you have more easily and getting ready to go out and tidying away become easier, too. A decluttered space equals a decluttered, clearer mind.

MAKE THAT CALL

Sending a text or an email is all well and good, and even the odd voice note (I am extremely partial to sending those), but it is not the same as picking up the phone to communicate properly with someone. Recognising their tone and knowing exactly how they are feeling can be much harder to do with text or email.

We live in a world where the art of conversation is dying, so pick up that phone, make that call and connect.

WHERE TO EAT

Be mindful: eat in a calm environment without too many distractions. TV dinners – of which I have had my fair share – aren't good for us. I mean, sure, you can do it every now and again, but don't make it a habit – not only because you're probably sitting hunched over, which is bad for digestion, but also because the noise and stimulation do not help the body with processing food. There is also a tendency to overeat in this situation, as you're not eating mindfully or slowly, and you can't always tell if you are full or not when you are not consciously in the moment, and so you just keep eating. I often find I am prone to snacking after a TV dinner, just consuming more without thought.

HYDRATION STATION

When you think you have drunk enough water, drink more. Hydration is key to good health and immunity, not to mention energy and glowing skin. Water hydrates the cells in our bodies, keeping us in tip-top condition. So get that goodness down you, and always carry a water bottle with you.

SMILE MORE

A big smile is not only infectious for all who see it, emitting positive energy, but it also uses fewer facial muscles than frowning. It's a no-brainer. It also tells the body that you are happy, signalling to the brain that all is OK, thus reducing stress. So, fake it to make it, and if in doubt, smile it out. I promise you, if you are in a funk, just grin to yourself and feel your mood shift.

LET YOURSELF BE LOVED

Open yourself up to feeling vulnerable. Take it from someone who had a closed heart for many, many years; not only was I closed to being loved, but I had no love for myself either. It is a sad waste of time. Life is short, so start working on that connection with yourself – open your heart up and see and feel the magic.

MASSAGE

The power of touch. Now, this might not be for everyone, but I personally adore a treatment. I love being touched, everywhere – be it a full-body treatment, foot reflexology, head, face, hands ... you name it, I'll take it!

The tension we hold in our bodies can cause so much discomfort. I have especially noticed more tension around my neck, along with headaches, since my forties. Perimenopause and menopause can cause frozen shoulder and headaches, as well as all sorts of other aches and pains, and I find treatments can help a lot.

Exercise is also brilliant, although it does create tighter muscles – something we all want, but they can tighten up too much and need to be rubbed down to ease the soreness.

Healing hands and a professional touch have immediate and long-term health and wellness benefits.

LAUGH FOR A MINUTE A DAY

At those times when I am feeling low or the lack of light due to the changing of the seasons in the UK or tiredness are getting to me, I try to laugh for a minute.

Now, this practice is grouped in the smile more and jump categories. When in a funk, try them all – they work.

Laughing releases stress and cannot fail to improve your mood, as well as being a good workout for your stomach muscles. Look in the mirror while you do it, as it is so bonkers it will literally crack you up. Time yourself for a minute.

WATER

Whether you swim in a pool, do wild swimming (if you can), shower or bathe, just get into some form of water each day. The healing powers of a good soak or rinse will soothe away aches and pains and wash away a bad day.

DO NOT PICK YOUR PIMPLES

As tempting as it is to try to take down the Mount Vesuvius that's started to erupt on your chin, don't do it. It will only make it angrier, and it will stick around for longer, looking unsightly, possibly getting infected and maybe even scarring. Instead, grab a piece of ice and apply it to the spot, which will bring down the inflammation.

MAKE MORE TIME FOR THE GOOD PEOPLE IN YOUR LIFE

Surround yourself with positive people – people who feed your soul, make you laugh and leave you feeling high on life.

BLURRED VISION

If you are starting to squint and these pages are getting blurry, get an eye test! Don't be vain – there are some great specs out there, so you will look gorgeous, I promise. Not wearing glasses or getting an eye test out of vanity or laziness will only cause more issues down the line, leading to headaches and dizziness. And those are possible symptoms of perimenopause and menopause anyway, so do yourself a favour and book that eye test.

TAKE A DEEP BREATH AND COUNT TO TEN

An oldie but a goodie. In times of extreme out-of-control moments, or if you feel you are getting angry or upset, just remember to take a deep breath to calm and centre yourself. You've got this!

DON'T LOSE YOUR CURIOSITY

Always stay curious about life and hold on to that desire to explore and find joy in the small things. Be more childlike in that innocent exploration; the inner child is still within every one of us. Reconnect and stop being so serious.

GET TO KNOW YOUR BODY

Our imperfections make us who we are. So, don't be afraid of your reflection; look at yourself, look at what makes you you. Don't shy away from looking at *all* of your body, taking a mirror and opening your legs and really looking at yourself. Don't be embarrassed or ashamed. It's your body; all bodies are beautiful, and all vaginas are unique and attractive in their own way.

THE GRASS ISN'T ALWAYS GREENER

I like to adopt the JOMO approach: the joy of missing out. How good does it feel to not make plans, stay home, have a bath, get some delicious food in, slide into your PJs, watch a film or finish reading that book? Once you have made the decision based on what you truly want to do, it's like a weight being lifted from your shoulders and the joy and contentment slowly warm you.

This is a feeling I aspire to, to be finally so happy with the power of saying no or cancelling. Or, better still, not making those plans in the first place – knowing instinctively that a night in or a weekend alone is what the doctor ordered.

GET YOUR CHECK-UPS

Go for your regular breast check-ups, blood tests or smear tests and keep on top of all health checks. Look out for moles, and if anything looks or feels strange to you about your body, go see a doctor to get it all looked at properly. Do not leave it – that is what the professionals are there for and we are so lucky in the UK with our National Health Service.

DO NOT RUN AWAY

We must face our fears and address them head on. This is something that I have had to learn the hard way, and it has taken a very long time.

LET'S BECOME OUR OWN TEACHERS

We all know in ourselves what feels good and what doesn't, so remember to follow that intuition – the signs are within you, always.

SING IN THE SHOWER

Be loud and proud and really enjoy releasing all the sound, however bad it might be. It makes a good start to the day and creates a happy endorphin release.

HAVE A BOOGIE

Whether you are cooking, brushing your teeth or in the shower, make sure that you have a little wiggle and shuffle throughout the day.

MAKE YOUR BED EVERY DAY

This may sound so simple, but the act of making your bed each morning will guarantee the best start. By doing this you accomplish your first task of the day; it's an instant win, which will give you a sense of pride and make you feel more productive and likely to continue with other tasks throughout the day.

LOOK AFTER YOUR TEETH

Go for regular hygienist check-ups. I try to go every six months. During perimenopause and menopause, our gums can become much more sensitive, even painful. I found that my teeth also moved, another side effect of the hormone changes, and I started to wear an Invisalign brace to help with this. If you are experiencing any problems like this, go to your dentist.

ALWAYS CARRY DENTAL FLOSS

This is something I always have with me in my handbag. I prefer those interdental brushes (the ones that look like mini pipe cleaners) – they're the best at getting bits of food out from between my teeth. This is another issue I have found with age. All not-so-sexy stuff. Ha!

LETTER TO MY YOUNGER SELF

Hey little Lisa,
This is an old friend who loves and cares for you very much.

I felt the need to check in with you and give you some advice as I know some days are harder than others and your confidence has been rocked because of the girls at school.

I know occasionally you feel lost and alone, but please don't let those bullies get to you. Jump on that BMX and ride as fast as you can towards an exciting future and a life full of adventures.

The main thing is, don't let it affect your confidence or let it make you fearful of people, or life. Not everyone is cruel or has bad intentions, even though right now it seems that way. If anything, I want you to be less afraid, to believe in yourself more and all you are capable of.

Dream big, little girl – whatever you wish for you can have. The world is your beautiful oyster.

Nurture that beautiful, creative mind you have, don't let yourself be sad too often.

Rise above it all and worry less, much less.

You've got this. I promise you.

You're going to have the most incredible life, that I can assure you ... Now, there will be some ups and downs – that we all know for sure – but the down times will make you appreciate all the good times there will be ... Cherish them.

You are going to have some wonderful people in your life, people that love you very much. Your family, for one, will always be endlessly proud of you; Nanna and Grandad couldn't love you more – hold them close, talk to them, confide in them, don't keep all that emotion to yourself.

I want you to have boundaries, to believe in your own self-worth, to realise what an incredible person you are. Be kind to everyone, be kind to yourself and always follow your intuition.

You will get this little pang in your tummy when you know that something isn't right for you. This is your body's way of telling you to stay safe, to stay guarded and maybe to stay away. It might be about people, it could be situations, but promise me you will listen to those signs – do not ignore them. This way you will be protected.

You will always have guardian angels around you, so trust in those signs, always.

You will make mistakes – that's life – but just try to learn along the way to not repeat them.

If you fail, pick yourself right back up again and realise that what isn't meant for you will pass you by and what is meant for you you will get in abundance.

Keep reading, lots; it brings you so much joy and will unlock huge creative potential within you and allow you to transport yourself into a beautiful fantasy world.

Write lots, too. Keep writing those diaries, your journals, and keep them so that you can read back over them in years to come. Never stop dancing, never stop singing – this is an expression of joy for you.

Do not let anyone intimidate you or make you think you are stupid. It is not true, and that will only hold you back. Everyone is learning at different speeds so take your time – there's so much to live for.

Keep enjoying the wonder and mystery of the moon and the stars and your crystals; this is going to become a very important part of your life.

Continue to find joy and wonder wherever you go, don't lose that free spirit and always continue to be that little loon – don't ever worry about fitting in ...

You won't always have all the answers, that may never happen. Just try to have a sense of self-awareness and an inner confidence to know that you are enough, so that when people try to put you down, you just walk away from them. Walk away from situations that do not serve you, and if for some reason you can't, learn quickly from them and don't repeat them.

Life is going to be full of fun, love and adventure. You will go on to do things that you only thought possible in your dreams and travel to the most wonderful places all around the world.

Grab life with both hands and jump right in.

All my love forever and ever,
Me xx

Useful Resources

Books

Frostrup, Mariella and Smellie, Alice, *Cracking the Menopause While Keeping Yourself Together* (Bluebird, 2021)

Harper, Dr Shahzadi and Bardwell, Emma, *The Perimenopause Solution: Take Control of Your Hormones Before They Take Control of You* (Vermilion, 2021)

Kaye, Dr Philippa, *The M Word: Everything You Need to Know About the Menopause* (Vie, 2023)

Mathews, Meg, *The New Hot: Taking on the Menopause with Attitude and Style* (Vermilion, 2020)

McCall, Davina and Potter, Dr Naomi, *Menopausing* (HQ, 2022)

For support and more information

British Menopause Society; https://thebms.org.uk/

Menopause Mandate; menopausemandate.com

Confidential advice, reassurance and education

womens-health-concern.org

wellbeingofwomen.org.uk

https://www.miscarriageassociation.org.uk/

References

1. Pilkington, S.M., Watson, R.E., Nicolaou, A., Rhodes, L.E. 'Omega-3 Polyunsaturated Fatty Acids: Photoprotective Macronutrients' *Experimental Dermatology* 2011 July 20(7):537–43. https://doi.org/10.1111/j.1600-0625.2011.01294.x

2. Li, J.N., Henning, S.M., Thames, G., *et al.*, 'Almond Consumption Increased UVB Resistance in Healthy Asian Women' *Journal of Cosmetic Dermatology* 2021; 20: 2975–2980. https://doi.org/10.1111/jocd.13946

3. Rybak, I., Carrington, A.E., Dhaliwal, S., Hasan, A., Wu, H., Burney, W., Maloh, J., Sivamani, R.K. 'Prospective Randomized Controlled Trial on the Effects of Almonds on Facial Wrinkles and Pigmentation' *Nutrients* 2021, *13*, 785. https://doi.org/10.3390/nu13030785

4. Stahl, W., Sies H. 'β-Carotene and Other Carotenoids in Protection from Sunlight' *The American Journal of Clinical Nutrition*, Volume 96, Issue 5, Nov 2012, 1179S–1184S. https://doi.org/10.3945/ajcn.112.034819

5. Scapagnini, G., Davinelli, S., Di Renzo, L., De Lorenzo, A., Olarte, H.H., Micali, G., Cicero, A.F., Gonzalez, S. 'Cocoa Bioactive Compounds: Significance and Potential for the

Maintenance of Skin Health' *Nutrients* 2014; 6(8):3202–3213. https://doi.org/10.3390/nu6083202

6. Guelinckx, I., Tavoularis, G., König, J., Morin, C., Gharbi, H., Gandy, J. 'Contribution of Water from Food and Fluids to Total Water Intake: Analysis of a French and UK Population Surveys' *Nutrients* 2016 Oct 14, 8(10):630. https://doi.org/10.3390/nu8100630

7. Penso, L., Touvier, M., Deschasaux, M., *et al.* 'Association Between Adult Acne and Dietary Behaviors: Findings from the NutriNet-Santé Prospective Cohort Study' *JAMA Dermatology* 2020;156(8): 854–862. https://doi.org/10.1001/jamadermatol.2020.1602

Acknowledgements

I commend anybody who talks about their journey openly but when I think back there were a couple of people who really stand out. One person who really shouted from the rooftops and pioneered this conversation was Meg Mathews. That woman singlehandedly spoke about everything. She released products available in all your local pharmacies and was everywhere talking about vaginal dryness and all the less pleasant symptoms others were afraid to talk about. That for me is truly remarkable, and I commend Meg for paving the way for us all. Meg has a fantastic book out, *The New Hot: Taking on the Menopause with Attitude and Style*, and she's done so much work in this space. I love and respect you, Meg – thank you for leading the way and for helping me. Mariella Frostrup is another woman who was talking openly on TV and in print years before anyone else bravely came forward and openly explored and shared information about this time in our lives.

Through both Meg and Mariella, I learned so much, and I would encourage you to check out Mariella's book, *Cracking the Menopause*, written alongside Alice Smellie. I would also like to thank the incredible women who are a part of the Menopause Mandate, a non-profit organisation campaigning for better support and help surrounding the menopause. I was asked by Mariella to be involved and I am proud to be a patron alongside Laura Biggs, Carolyn Harris MP and her team, Davina McCall, Gabby Logan, Penny Lancaster, Dr Shahzadi Harper and Michelle Griffith-Robinson, to name but a few.

Huge thanks to Dr Naomi Potter, who has become a close friend over the last few years – she is a fount of knowledge and a continued inspiration. I am learning more and more about female health challenges and Hormone Replacement Therapy every week on our live Instagram series, 'Midweek Menopause Madness'.

I was lucky enough to be able to include in this book advice from my brilliant expert friends: Dr Charlotte Gooding, Paul Webb, Emma Bardwell, Dr Megan Rossi, Rhiannon Lambert and Dr Naomi Potter.

I am honestly so grateful to the gorgeous friends who read and said nice things about the book, and to the ladies in my life, who are always there standing by the side lines: Michele, Zoe, Lucy, and Jules, one of my biggest supporters for the longest time, championing me from afar.

I'd also like to thank my team: Katie, Richard, Emily and Madison at M&C Saatchi. I love you all, and I'm so grateful to have you in my corner.

Thank you to the HarperCollins team, especially to Ajda, my editor, who believed in me from the beginning – your enthusiasm and encouragement was unfaltering. To Georgina, Hannah, Isabel, Caroline, Holly and the wider team – thank you so much for your help and guidance.

To my beautiful family; my dad Nigel, my mum Lydia and my two sisters, Lesley-Ann and Joanna, I'm so grateful for you all and I love you very much. And, of course, my George … Thank you for always being there. I love you.

To the women who have come before us, the women who didn't have the information, the love, advice and support we are lucky enough to have now that this conversation has become louder – women like my Nanna Nora, the warrior matriarch who left the biggest impression on me, who I miss every day. I will always love and respect you and admire you more than you will ever know.

And finally, to my niece Willow. I hope one day you will read this book, and not make the mistakes I have made, with these lessons in life, love and menopause.